In The Season Thereof

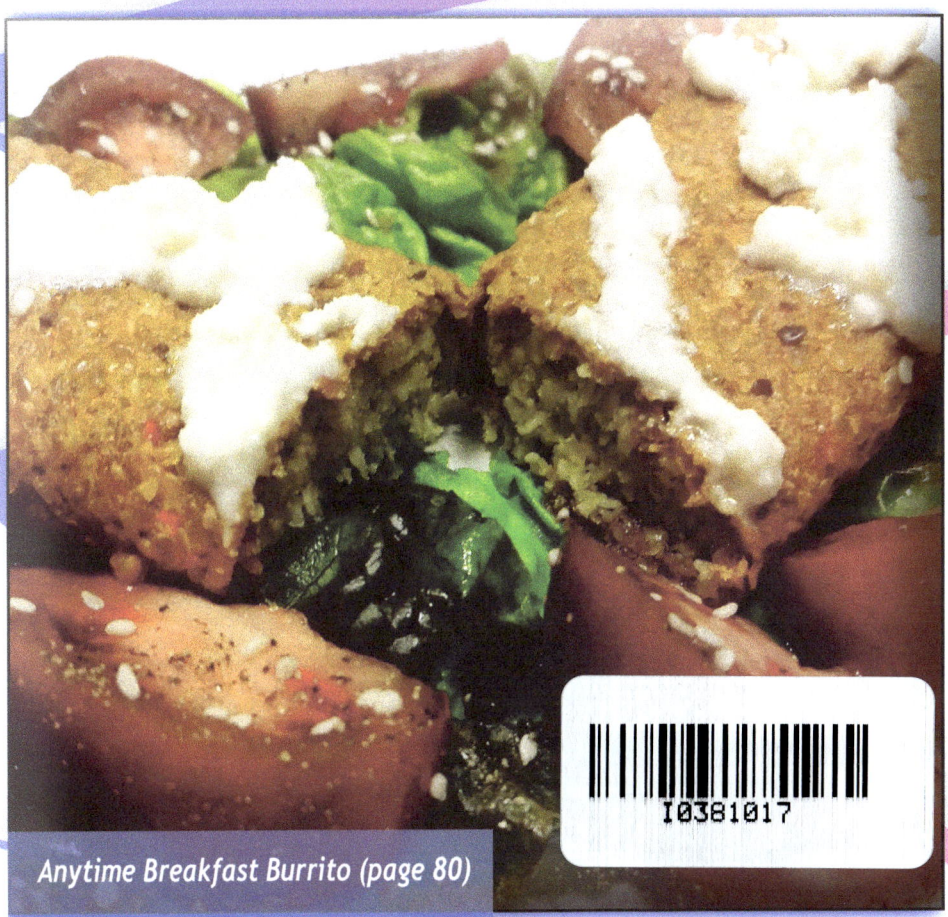

Anytime Breakfast Burrito (page 80)

Simple gourmet plant based raw food recipes

By Kachina Choate
Summer Bear

In the Season Thereof
Simple gourmet plant based raw food recipes
Copyright © 2020 Kachina Choate

All rights reserved. No part of this publication may be reproduced, stored in a retrieval system, or transmitted in any form or by any means, electronic, mechanical, photocopying, recording, or otherwise, without the prior written consent of the copyright owner.
dollkachina@gmail.com

First Edition 2004 Second Edition 2020

ISBN 978-1-938142-04-8 (print)
ISBN 978-1-938142-05-5 (ebook)

1. Raw Foods 2. Cookery (Natural foods) 3. Vegetarian Food

This book does not intend to cure or give medical advice. We want to educate, inform, and empower readers to make their own decisions on their health and well-being. Each person might have different reactions to changes in diet. If you have concerns about your health or nutrition, consult your healthcare advisor.

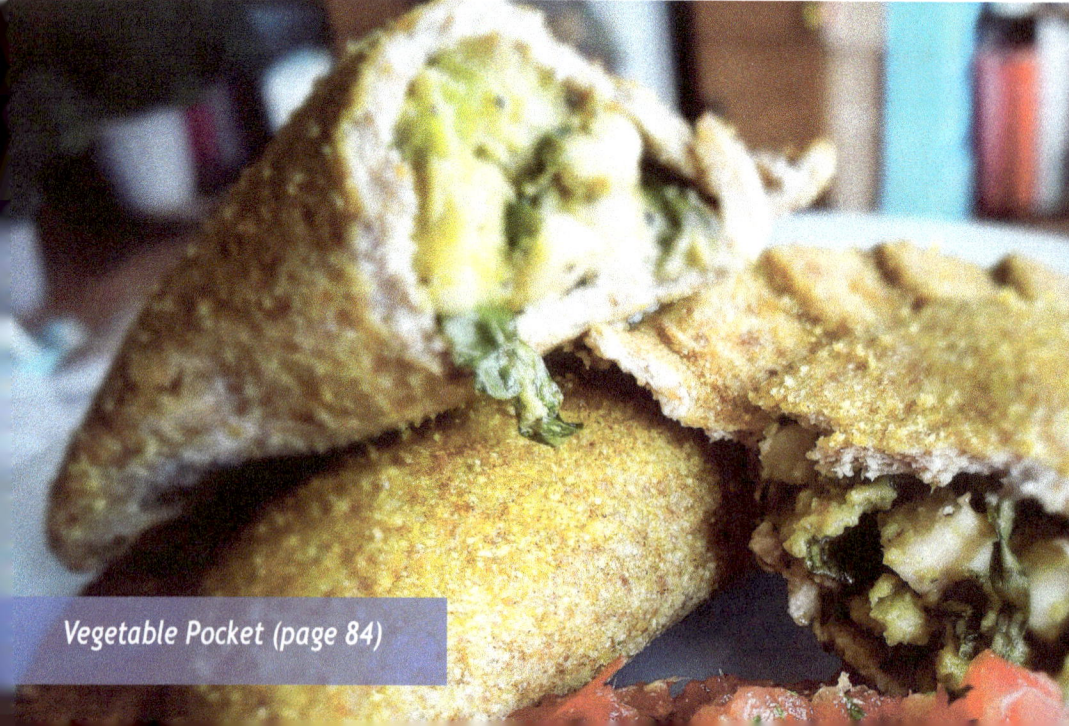

Vegetable Pocket (page 84)

CONTENTS

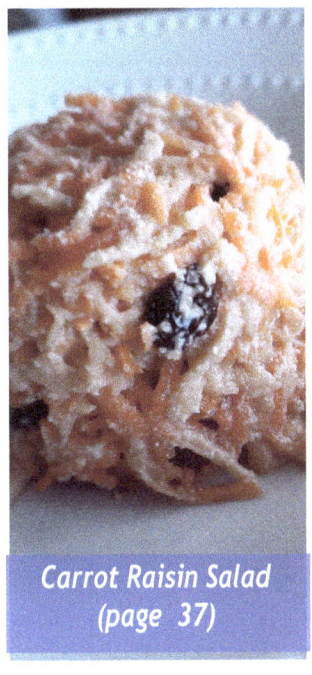

Carrot Raisin Salad (page 37)

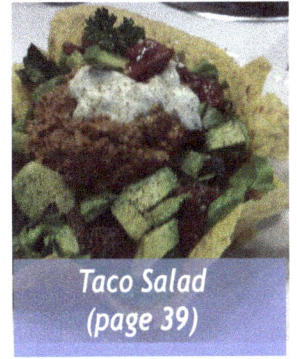

Taco Salad (page 39)

Basil Citrus Juice (page 22)

4
INTRODUCTION

5
IN THE SEASONS

6
MENU PLANNING

7
BASIC FOOD STORAGE

16
BEVERAGES

26
SOUPS & SALADS

53
SIDE & MAIN DISHES

98
DESERTS

130
BREAD

142
NON-DAIRY

150
MISCELLANEOUS

153
APENDIX

155
INDEX

159
SEASONAL RECIPE INDEXES

Introduction

When I began eating natural raw foods in 2002, people would ask, "Don't you get tired of just eating salads?" The answer was yes. I was missing some of my old favorite foods and getting bored of the recipes that were available at the time. That is why I started creating recipes.

After a while and a few potlucks, people started asking, "How do you make that wonderful food?" The answer it took practice and learning new skills.

At first, I had a hard time thinking how to make raw foods, it just didn't make sense to me. I went to demos and classes, but by the time I got home I would have no idea how to prepare the food. Even though I had been cooking for years, it took my friend Karie walking me though every step of a recipe down to cut avocado and remove the pit, before it clicked. Ever since then I have been having fun playing with food.

Food should be fun and taste good. Don't be afraid to experiment. Some of my favorite recipes are made from leftovers.

Take this chance, be the chef. It may not be easy at first but with practice you can do it.

I recommend that you keep a notebook and pen in the kitchen, so you can write down the recipes you create, or you can be like my friend, Sarah, who said, "Are you enjoying eating this? Good, because you won't get it again. I don't remember how I made it."

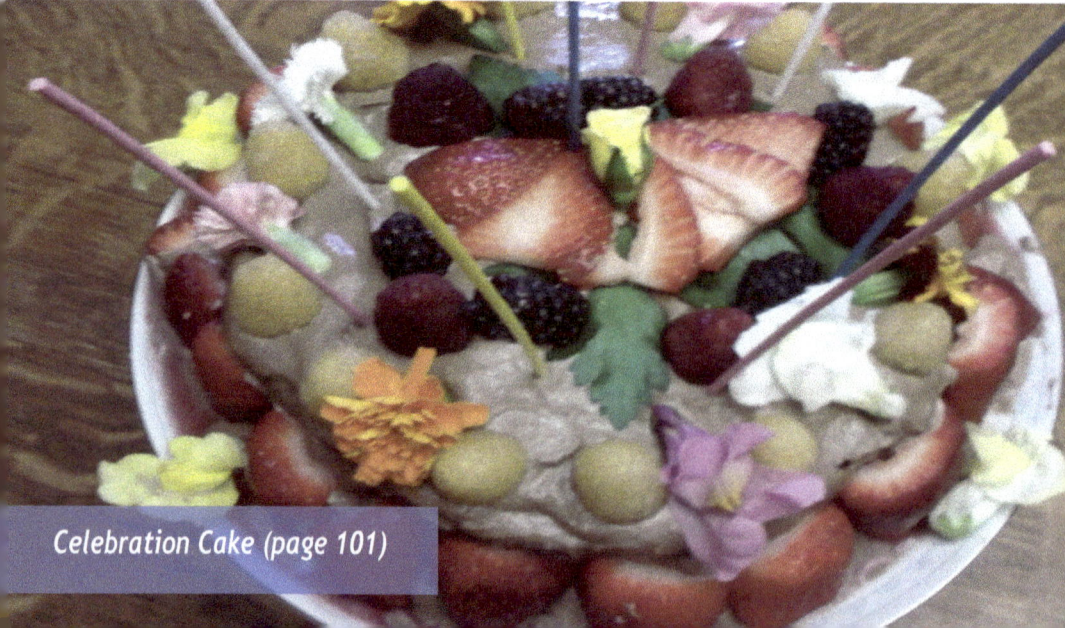

Celebration Cake (page 101)

In The Season Thereof

*To everything there is a season,
and a time to every purpose
under the heaven:
A time to be born,
and a time to die;
a time to plant,
and a time to pluck up
that which is planted;*

Ecclesiastics 3:1-2

Foods eaten in season are fresher and have higher nutrition; they are better for your body and usually less expensive. Usually the produce on sale are the ones in season where it was grown. It is also an easy way to support your local farmers and economy.

Think food has the same nutrition year-round? A 1997 research study in England found significant differences in the nutrient content of pasteurized milk in the summer versus winter. Iodine was higher in the winter, whereas beta-carotene was higher in the summer. These differences in milk composition were primarily due to differences in the diets of the cows.

Similar research in Japan found a threefold difference in vitamin C content of spinach harvested in summer versus winter.

The point is that eating food in season not only taste better, it has more nutrition. Seasonal eating also helps the body prepares for the coming season.

Spring is a time for the body to recover from winter and prepare for summer heat. Common spring foods include leafy greens, tender vegetables, berries, and fruit.

Summer is hot and provides a bounty of cooling foods to help us withstand heat. Summer foods include: melons, vegetables, fruits, dark green leafy vegetables, and herbs.

Fall is a time of bounty and preparing for the cold winter months head. Apples, pears, tubers, and starchy vegetables are plentiful. As it gets cooler, it is also a time to include the warming spices such as ginger, peppercorns, and mustard seeds in the diet.

Winter is cold, and time to eat more warming foods. Generally, foods that take longer to grow are more warming than foods that grow quickly. Good winter foods include root vegetables, seeds, grains, nuts, and sprouts. Many times, during the cold months, growing sprouts may be the only source of fresh greens.

While I have tried to place the recipes in the correct season, some of the food crosses seasons. In those cases, I placed it in the season I thought made since, but you can decide when you want to eat it. There are a few items that, while they can be made in any season, I placed in the one that it is traditionally eaten in.

> *The difference between fair food and great food is how it is spiced. The great thing about making your own food is that you can spice it how you like it. For example, if you want more or less salt then adjust it.*

Steps to Menu Planning

1. Look through your favorite recipes.
2. Write out what will you be eating for breakfast, lunch, dinner, and snacks for the week.

   Note: When you're doing this step, it is a good thing to look at the calendar to see what appointments and events you have during the week and make your meal plans accordingly. On busy days plan simple food, and on days you have time to prepare, then plan more gourmet food.

3. Prepare a grocery list. I have found when I have a list, I save money even if I don't eat everything that I plan.

Menu Ideas

When beginning to transition to a new diet, people often want ideas of what to eat. One way is to use menus.

Have no idea of what to put on a menu? I suggest that you look at converting menus you currently use and adapting them to your new diet. For example, think about lasagna. It is traditionally served with salad and garlic bread. I might make:

Menu 1

Zucchini Lasagna (page 76)
Garlic Bread (page 147)
Green Salad with Italian Dressing (page 52)

It also helps to have a list of what you have in your pantry when making a menu. If you have something that needs to be rotated, use it in the plan. This also helps you know what needs to be replaced.

Menu 2

Eggless Salad
(page 34)
Baykon
(page 87)
Carrot Juice

Menu 3

Party Dip
(page 53)
Flax Crackers
(page 139)
Banana Date
Kebabs (page 129)

Menu 4

Vegetable pocket
(page 84)
Dirty Rice
(page 69)
Fresh Fruit

Menu 5

Green Vegetable Salad
Peach Mint Lemonade
(page 20)
Lemon Pie
(page 108)

Menu 6

Brazil Nut Burger
(page 74)
Spicy Jicama Fries
(page 64)
Frosty Drink
(page 19)

Menu 7

Middle Eastern
Marinated Eggplant
(page 78)
Lemon Rice
(page 67)
Tomatoes with Basil

Basic Food Storage Ideas

Many people think you can't fallow a raw food diet when you need to rely on food storage. Nuts, seeds, and grains used for making cheese, milk, bread, sweets and other raw food are good for storage. Add dried, freeze-dried fruit and vegetables, and sprouting seeds for source of fresh food.

When making blender soup I make double batch, take half of it and dry it on non-stick dehydrator sheet like fruit leather. When completely dry, powder it in coffee grinder, label it and you have instant soup mix, all you need to do is add water. I not only use this for my food storage but when I don't feel like preparing dinner or when camping or hiking.

Once you have food, it may be nice to have tools to help prepare it. Some tools I suggest are sprouting equipment, manual wheatgrass juicer, spiralizer for noodles, tortilla press for dough, dehydrator (a sun dryer or car window will work).

Other items that help are a mortar and pestle for grinding nuts and seeds. Look through the stores and see if they have manual equipment that you would use. Some items to think about purchasing include a manual wheat grinder, a manual food processor and blender. I have seen blender bikes and hand cranked ones. Use them before they are needed. In this way, you will know how they work and how easy it is to clean.

I strongly suggest that you try to live off your food storage for a week or two to see if you are storing what you need. Look through your recipe books and see what could be made out of your food storage.

For more information on food storage and recipes using food storage look for Thriving on Plant Based Food Storage Raw food recipes featuring dried fruits and vegetables by Kachina Choate of Summer Bear.

Grains:

All grains should be whole and have the ability to sprout.

wheat berries,
kamut, or spelt
oat groats
buckwheat
barley
rye
quinoa
others

Seeds:

black wild rice
flax
sesame
sunflower
pumpkin
poppy

Sprouting Seeds:

fenugreek
broccoli
alfalfa
cabbage
sunflower
radish
others

Dried & Freeze Dried Fruits:

dates
raisins
figs
apples
apricots
pineapple
pears
banana
papaya
mango
strawberries
peaches
coconut

Any other fruits that appeal to you. I dry almost everything when it is in season and store it.

Dried & Freeze Dried Vegetables:

tomatoes *(my experience is that I have never have enough dried tomatoes)*
peas
corn
green beans
zucchini
variety of squash
mushrooms
onions
celery
cabbage
spinach
kale
garlic
powdered green drink
others

Store root vegetables, such as onions, garlic, cabbage, carrots, and apples in a root cellar for the following year when they are in season. Do not store apples with other items!

Nuts:

almonds
walnuts
pecans
cashews
brazil nuts
pine nuts
macadamia
others

Oils:
(Be srue to rotate these!)

olive
flax

any coldpressed oil you like

food grade essential oils *(lemon, grapefuit, cinnamomon, ginger, lime, oragne, pepperment, etc...)*

Sweeteners:

raw honey
raw agave
raw coconut nectar
raw coconut sugar
dates
raisins
other dried fruit

Seasonings:
(Store what you use)

raw carob
cayenne pepper
pepper corns (with grinder)
Himalayan crystal salt
ginger
garlic powder
onion powder
curry
turmeric
celery seed
mustard seed
cloves
chili powder
marjoram
sage
rosemary
thyme
alum
cream of tartar
basil
parsley
lemon peel
lime peel
orange peel
Mexican season
chili seasoning
Italian seasoning
pumpkin pie seasoning
poultry seasoning

Introducing the family

More than once I have been asked "how do I make my family eat raw foods?" The answer no one wants to hear is you cannot make them do anything.

Be patient and don't force. My mom, not a picky eater as a child tasted clam chowder at school and didn't like it. When she was going to dump the tray, her teacher said she couldn't leave until ate it all. The teacher stood over her and used fear to force her to eat it. My mom ate it with tears rolling down her cheeks and clam chowder going down in lumps. The teacher was very pleased with herself until the chowder came back up all over her shoes. That was the first and last time my mom ever ate clam chowder.

Don't let food become a power struggle. I believe in the importance of choice. You are more likely to receive a lot of resistance if you command your family to eat a new diet.

I have found the more I pushed someone to eat my way, the more that person resists. But when I asked them to taste it and used some of the following tips, they became more and more willing to eat new food and even began to enjoy what I made.

Allow older children and spouses the freedom to choose what they wish to eat. I have found that if you get children involved in making food, they are more likely to try it. My little 4-year-old neighbor came over and helped me prepare a meal. He was so excited to actually be in the kitchen making food. When the meal was complete, he sat down with his fork and spoon, enthusiastic to try his creation. He tasted it, got a funny look on his face, tasted it again, and said, "I don't like it." The point is that while he didn't like that meal, he had fun in the kitchen and continued to help make other meals that he did like.

It may be helpful to practice the Law of Substitution. When you take something away from your family, give them something in return. Some examples might be:

- Take away refined sugar, and replace it with a natural sweetener such as fresh fruit, sweets made with raw honey, agave nectar, or coconut nectar.

- Replacing salty store chips with natural homemade kale chips, flax crackers, or nuts that have been soaked overnight in Himalayan Crystal salt and dried, crunchy vegetables especially organic celery.

- Drinking fresh fruit and vegetable juices instead of soda.

Supplying the Kitchen

Having some essential equipment and knowledge will help make your preparation whole lot less stressful. For your convenience, I have provided suggested equipment.

- **Knives, Cutting Boards, Bowls, and Pans:** choose ones that you love.

- **Food processor:** is the 1st piece I would buy. It becomes your new best friend, and I use it almost every day. Choose one that has a lot of power.

- **Blender:** the most powerful blender you can afford. Even ones that do not have 1000 W of power will work for your food; it just may not be as creamy or fluffy as the more powerful blenders.

- **Dehydrator:** the brand does not really matter as long as it has a temperature control. I prefer the box type dehydrators with removable trays, this makes it easier to make pies, cakes, and casseroles.

- **Nonstick dehydrator sheets:** flexible sheets used with dehydrators.

- **Sprouting equipment:** I have the best success using the tray method. Get equipment that works the best for you.

- **Spiral slicer:** a vegetable slicer used to make vegetable noodles.

- **Juicer:** if you want to make nut butters and banana ice cream, then you will need to get a masticating type juicer.

Don't worry about getting equipment all at one time. Start with what you will use the most. I already had knives, so the first tool I purchased was a food processor. I used my old blender until I could afford the one I wanted.

Definitions

Some common terms used in raw food preparation include:

Enzyme = produced by a living organism and functions as a biochemical catalyst. It helps regulate chemical reactions throughout the lifespan of the organism.

Enzyme inhibitor = molecules that binds to enzymes and decreases their activity.

Raw Food = food that is raw, not cooked. Some products that are not raw because of the temperature in which they were processed including: balsamic vinegar, bulgur wheat, couscous, pasteurized juice etc.

Living Food = food that is freshly picked directly from the plant and is eaten immediately or prepared in a way (such as soaking nuts or sprouting) to activate enzymes.

Whole Foods Plant-Based (WFPB) = a way of eating that emphasizes whole plants including vegetables, fruits, whole grains, legumes, seeds and nuts. This would include vegan and raw food diets.

Whole Foods Plant-Based, No Oil (WFPBNO) = is a version of whole food plant-based diet but excludes all oil.

Transition Food = Food that is used to transition from traditional standard diet to a raw food diet. Some transition foods include: maple syrup (grade B or C), molasses (it has been heated) and gourmet raw foods. Some people use bottled ketchup, tofu, veganinase, and sugar; these products are not raw. When going to potlucks, I recommend that you don't use them.

Superfoods = Food that is nutrient rich and beneficial for health. Superfoods include: walnuts, Brussels sprouts, acai berries, cacao, avocadoes etc.

Raw Liquid Sweetener = includes, but may not be limited to, coconut nectar, agave nectar, raw honey (vegans don't eat honey) etc.

When I started it helped me to think about the way I made food in the following conversions:

> Food Preparation = cook
> Fry = warm, no greater than 110 degrees
> Boil = soak
> Cook = prepare
> Bake = dehydrate

When most raw food recipes call for nuts, they mean soaked nuts, unless otherwise stated; hard nuts like almonds 12-24 hours, soft nuts 4-6 hours. After nuts have been soaked, the enzymes are active, and nuts will spoil if not used in a day or two. Keep them refrigerated after soaking.

Sprouting

Sprouting happens when a seed germinates and begins to grow. Sprouts are considered living foods.

Energy is released and natural chemical changes occur so they are easier for the human body to assimilate. They are a convenient way to have fresh vegetables in any season and are easily grown in your home.

There are many methods of sprouting (jar, paper-towel, and tray). All sprouting is started by soaking seeds overnight, then placing the seeds in a jar or tray. Water seed two times a day. Drain water completely. The sprouts are ready when they start growing tails (1 to 6 days). Rinse and drain sprouts every three days after harvesting and store in the refrigerator, they keep up to a week.

Some sprouts can be grown into tender green plants (microgreens) such as peas, sunflower, and kale.

Note: Some bean sprouts such as pinto beans are very bitter when eaten raw. If using pinto beans, sprout them and then lightly steam them to remove bitterness.

Sprouts from nightshade family such as tomatoes, potatoes, peppers, and eggplants should not be eaten as the sprouts are toxic.

Sprouting Rice

Wild rice is not really rice it is the seed of an aquatic grass. There are four species of wild rice. One native to Asia it is harvested as a vegetable. The other three are found in the Great Lakes region and harvested as grains.

Black wild rice will sprout, or bloom, by soaking it in water and changing water daily. This differs from other sprouts because rice grows in water.

Soak 1-2 cups of rice in water overnight. Drain and rinse and add fresh water. Rinse rice every day keeping rice covered in water 2-6 days (the length of sprouting time may vary based on climactic factors). Rice is ready to eat when it is soft and easy to chew, some wild black rice will split down the middle.

Brown rice can be sprouted but does not taste very good in my opinion. White rice will not sprout as the germ has been removed.

Note: quinoa will sprout like wild rice in water.

Drying Nuts & Seeds

After soaking nuts and seeds to release the enzyme inhibitors, I like to dehydrate ones I am not using in a recipe right away. Once nuts are soaked, they will spoil. By drying them, they keep for a longer time and they are ready to use when needed. Dehydrate them at 100° F for about 18 hours.

> **Fun Facts**
>
> *An enzyme inhibitor is a molecule that binds to enzymes and decreases their activity. They are nature's way of preserving and making nuts, seeds, and grains last for a long period of time.*

Salt

There are enormous differences between standard, refined table salt and natural salt. Table salt is manufactured salt that is stripped of its natural minerals. Salt is not a dangerous food, however, the in the process of refining table salt sodium becomes out of balance and other minerals are lost. To keep salt from clumping anti-caking agents are added. One of the most common contain aluminum.

You don't have to eliminate salt entirely just refined table salt. Choose natural unrefined salt. These salts retain minerals other than just sodium that are good for the body.

Sea salt is a better option but be careful as 89% of all sea salt producers now refine their salt. Sea salt is not quite as healthy as it used to be. Remember that our oceans are being used as dumping grounds for harmful toxic poisons.

My preferred salt is Himalayan crystal salt (it is pink in color).

The Fresenius Institute in Europe analyzed Himalayan crystal salt and found that it has an amazing array of important trace minerals and elements including; potassium, calcium and magnesium. These minerals help your body achieve balance by restoring fluids and replenishing your supply of electrolytes when sweating heavily.

Celtic salt is another popular unrefined salt and is grayish in color.

Real salt (Redmond) is unrefined and the only pink salt and mined in America.

Olive Oil

"Expeller Pressed" is a continuous feed method where oil is squeezed from the raw material in one step under high pressure. All cold pressed oil is expeller pressed, but not all expeller pressed oil is cold pressed.

If the bottle says expeller pressed, it may or may not have been processed under high heat. The only way to know for sure is to call the manufacturer or if the label clearly states "cold pressed".

Olive Oil Labeling

Olive oil labeling can be confusing, here is a list of terms you may see.

Extra-virgin olive oil (EVOO) comes from the first pressing of olives, contains no more than 0.8% acidity, and is judged to have a superior taste. There can be no refined oil in extra-virgin olive oil.

Virgin olive oil has an acidity less than 2% acidity and is judged to have a good taste. There can be no refined oil in virgin olive oil.

Olive oil is a blend of virgin oil and refined virgin oil, containing at most 1% acidity. It commonly lacks a strong flavor.

Olive-pomace oil is a blend of refined pomace olive oil and possibly some virgin oil. It is fit for consumption, but it may not be called olive oil. Olive-pomace oil is rarely found in a grocery store; it is often used for certain kinds of cooking in restaurants.

Lampante oil is olive oil not used for consumption; lampante comes from olive oil's ancient use as fuel in oil-burning lamps. Lampante oil is mostly used in the industrial market.

Beware of oil blends labeled as olive oil.

Chamomile Lemonade

Preparation: 10 Min.　　Chilling: 1-2 Hrs.　　Makes 4-6 Servings

Ingredients

- 5 apples
- 4 lemons
- 5 tbsp. chamomile or 6 bags chamomile tea
- 1 c. pure water
- lemon slices, for garnish

Directions

Place chamomile and water in a glass jar. Cover and place in the sun for 30 to 60 minutes.

Peel and juice apples and lemons. Strain out the chamomile or remove the tea bags. Mix juice with tea.

Serve in a glass that has been chilled and top with a slice of lemon for garnish.

Fun Fact

Traditionally, chamomile is thought to promote better sleep, soothe stomach problems, menstrual cramps, and hemorrhoids. Growing chamomile in a garden not only adds to the appearances of the garden it can be very useful. It facilitates growth of the surrounding plants and even heals nearby sick plants.

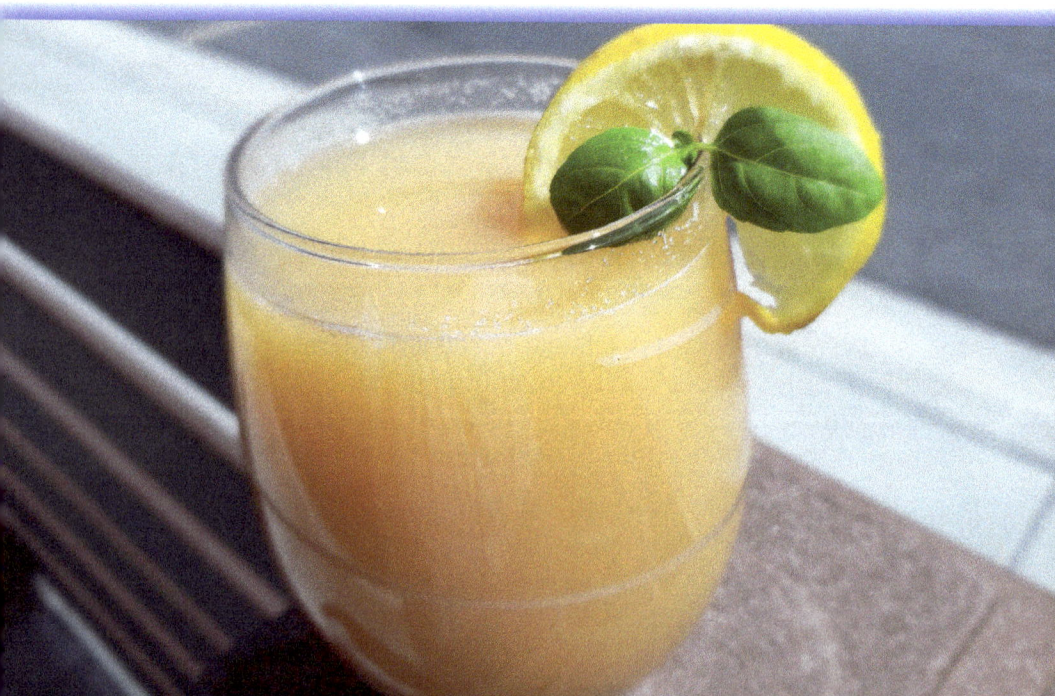

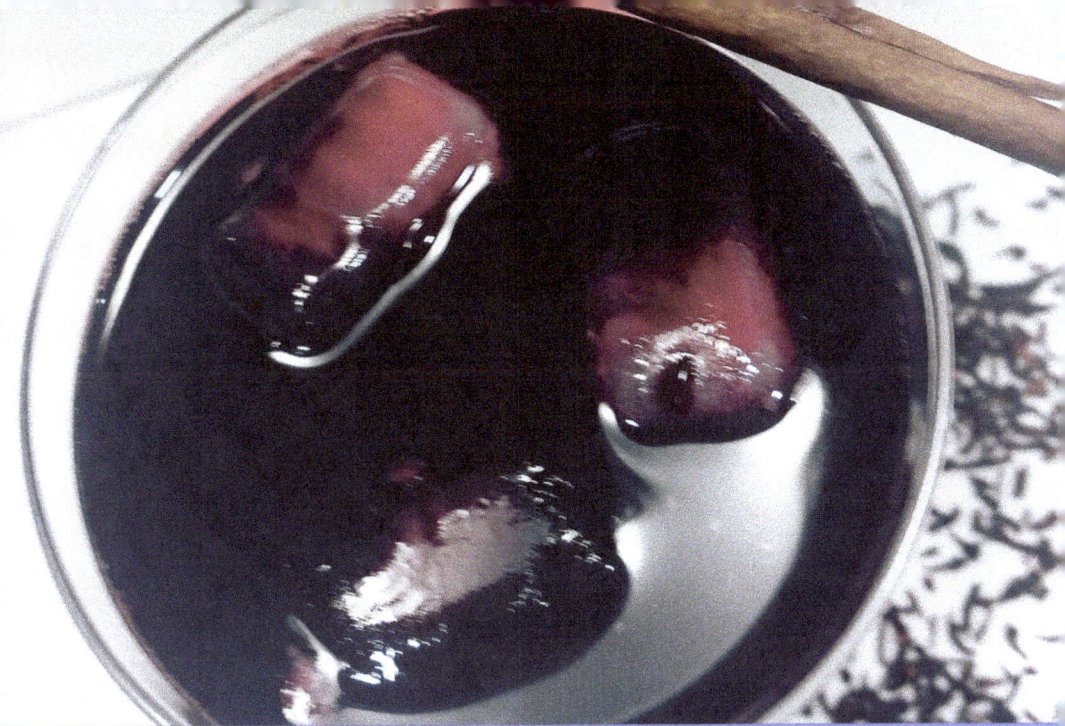

Hibiscus Drink

Preparation: 10 Min.   Chilling: 1-2 Hrs.   Makes 6-8 Servings

Ingredients

- ½ c. dried hibiscus flowers
- 1 four-inch cinnamon stick
- 10 whole cloves
- ¼ tsp. allspice, crushed
- 6-inch piece fresh ginger, or 1 tbsp. dried
- 4 apples, juiced
- 5 c. water
- ½ c. raw liquid sweetener (optional)

Directions

In a glass jar, place pure water, dried hibiscus flowers, cinnamon stick, cloves, crushed allspice, and ginger. Set in the hot sun for 4 to 6 hours.

Juice apples. Strain the hibiscus liquid into a pitcher; add the apple juice, and chill.

This is a tangy drink. If you would like it sweeter, add as much raw sweetener as needed. Serve drink over ice, use a hibiscus flower or cinnamon stick as garnish.

Fun Fact

In Mexico, dried hibiscus is a delicacy. The Roselle hibiscus is commonly used as a vegetable and is a common ingredient in chicken soup in the Visayan Islands.

Mint Shake

Preparation: 10 Min.   Makes 2-4 Servings

Ingredients

- 1 c. fresh mint
- ¼ c. coconut nectar
- 1 c. macadamia or cashew nuts
- 1 tbsp. lemon juice
- 1 c. water
- crushed ice cubes

Directions

In a blender, place coconut nectar, macadamia nuts, lemon juice and water mix until smooth.

Reserve a few sprigs of mint for garnish. Add the reaming mint and pulse until the drink is specked with tiny green flecks.

Crush ice cubes and place in a glass. Pour the drink over the ice and garnish with mint.

Fun Fact

Mint is a symbol of hospitality and wisdom used by ancient Hebrews who scattered min on synagogue floors so footsteps would release its fragrance.

Mango Smoothie

Preparation: 10 Min.   Makes 2-4 Servings

Ingredients

- ½ mango
- 1 banana
- 1 large orange
- 2 tsp. chia seeds
- 1 tbsp. sesame seeds
- 3 tsp. coconut nectar
- ½ c. water

Directions

Wash and peel mango. Cut the flesh off the pit, place mango in blender, though away the pit. Break peeled banana into small pieces add to blender.

Place just squeezed orange juice along with chia seeds, sesame seeds, and coconut nectar with mango blend until smooth. Add water as needed or until desired thickness is achieved. The drink should be very smooth and creamy.

Pour into glasses and serve. Garnish with slice of orange or mango.

Fun Fact

The oldest known mango tree is 300 years old and still produces viable fruit, located in East Khandesh

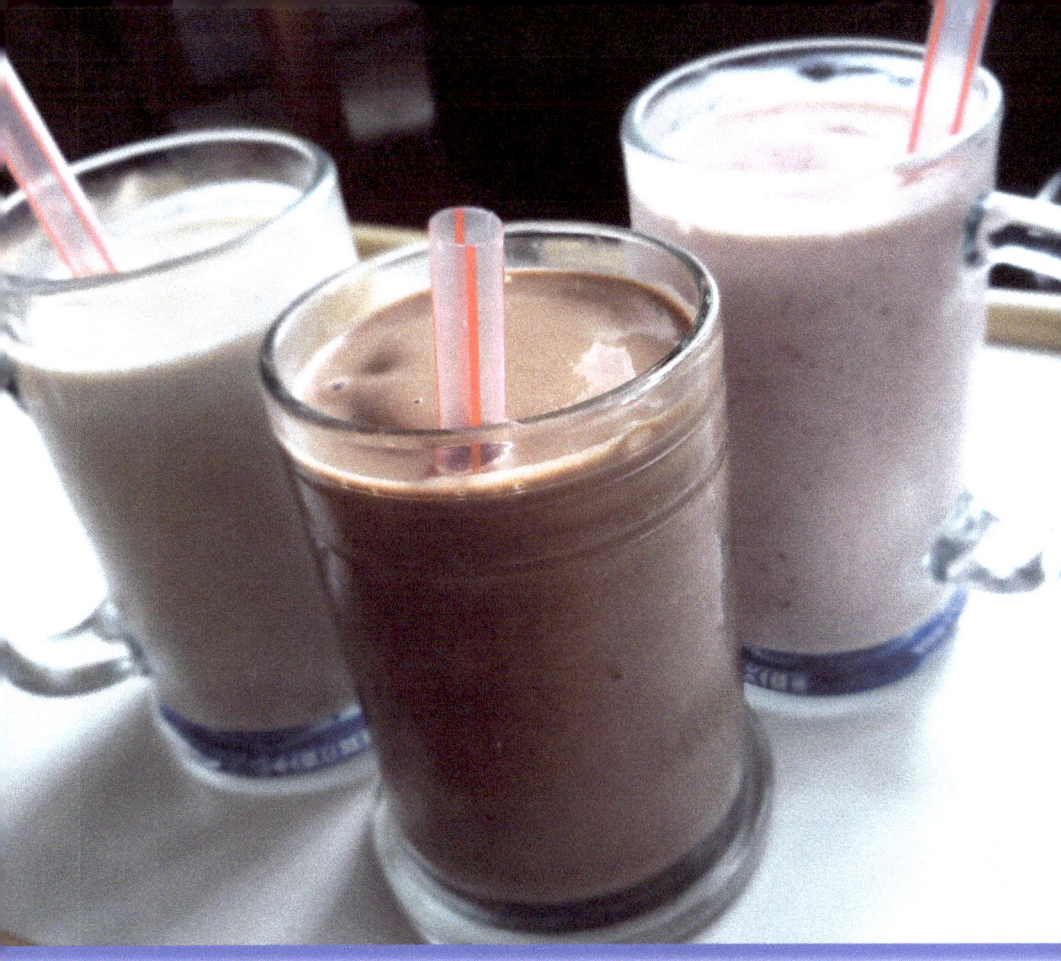

Frosty Drink

Preparation: 5 Min.

Makes 6-8 Servings

Ingredients

- 2 c. sesame seed milk (page 142)
- 2-4 bananas, frozen
- ¼ c. raw liquid sweetener
- 4 tbsp. raw carob powder

Directions

Use bananas that have been peeled then frozen. Place bananas in a blender along with sesame milk, honey, carob, and strawberries.

Blend until it is thick and smooth. Pour into a glass and enjoy.

Variations

1) For a strawberry frosty, omit carob and add strawberries.

2) For vanilla frosty, omit carob, add 2 inches vanilla bean or 2 teaspoons raw vanilla powder.

Peach Mint Lemonade

Preparation: *Chilling:*   *Makes 2-4*
15 Min.   1-2 Hrs.   Servings

Ingredients

- 4 fresh peaches
- 4 medium lemons
- 3 medium apples
- ½ c. raw liquid sweetener (optional)
- 1 tbsp. fresh mint
- 1 ½ c. pure water

Directions

Peel peaches, lemons and apples, discard pits and seeds. Juice peaches, lemons and apples along with fresh mint.

In a large bowl combine the juice, sweetener if desired, and water. Pour into glass over ice and garnish with a sprig of mint.

Fun Fact

Many Hindu cultures believe that basil is favored by the gods and therefore is sacred. In other places, basil is seen by young couples as a sign of love and devotion.

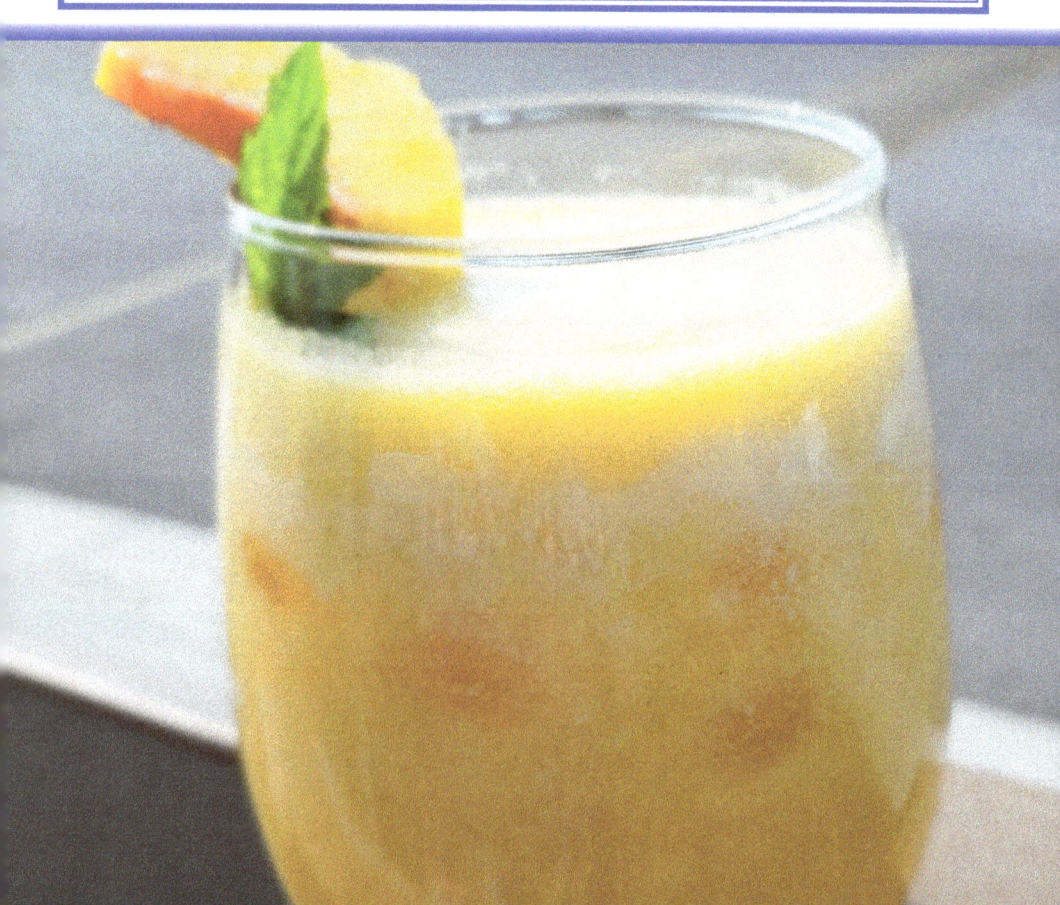

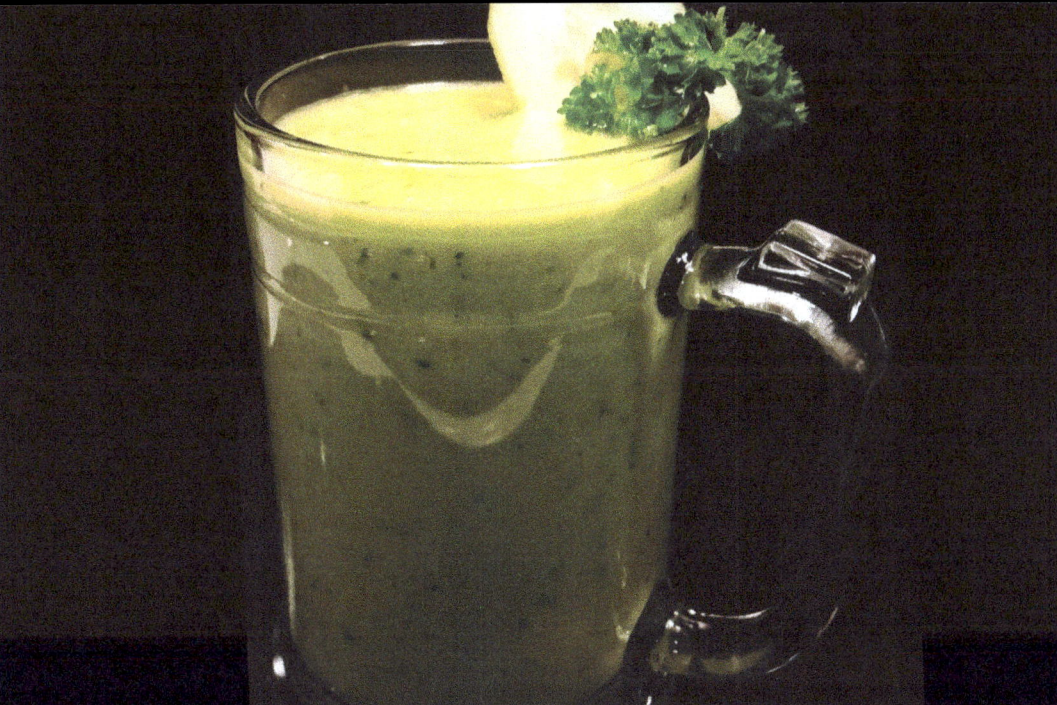

Mexican Mind Meld

Preparation: 10 Min.

Makes 2-4 Servings

Ingredients

- 1 large cucumber, peeled
- 1 avocado
- ½ c. fresh parsley
- 2 green onions
- ½ jalapeno pepper, seeded
- 1 clove garlic
- 1 celery stalk
- 2 c. hemp seed milk (page 142)

Directions

Make hempseed milk. Cut jalapeno and remove seeds.

In a blender, combine peeled cucumber, avocado that has been peeled and pit removed, green onions, jalapeno pepper, garlic, celery, and hemp seed milk.

Purée until very smooth. Serve in a chilled glass, preferably a tall one. Garnish with parsley sprigs.

Variation

Other nut or seed milks can be used in place of hemp seed milk.

Fun Fact

Jalapenos help lower blood pressure and fight migraine headaches. They also happened to be the first peppers to go into space on a NASA shuttle.

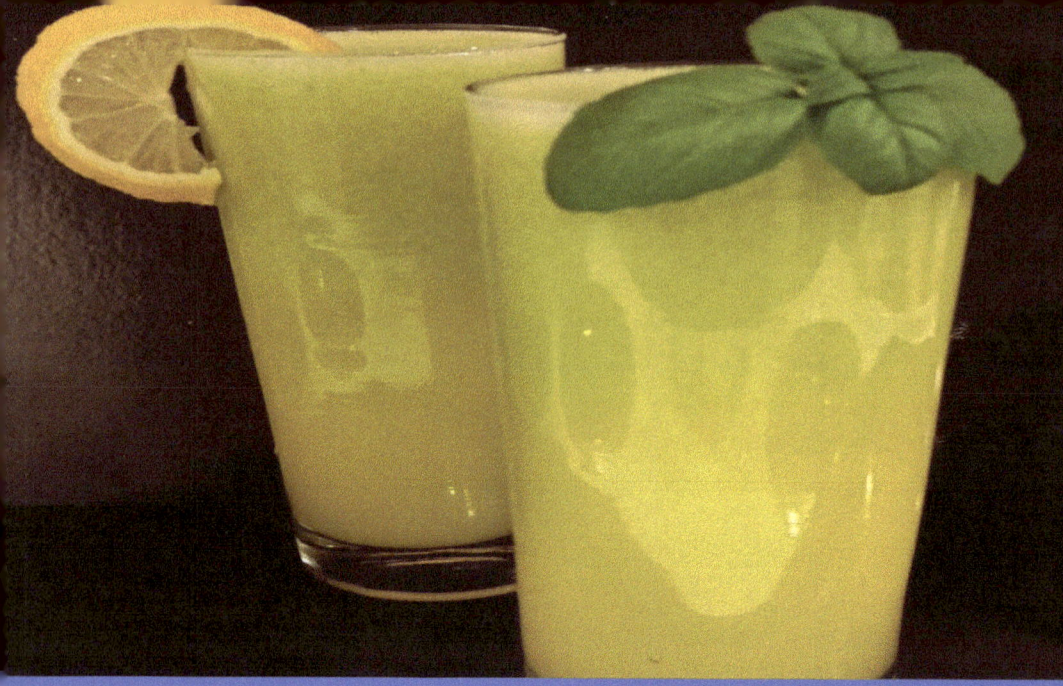

Basil Citrus Juice

Preparation: 10 Min.   Chilling: 1-2 Hrs.   Makes 4-6 Servings

Ingredients

- ½ c. fresh basil
- 5 limes, juiced
- 2 lemons, juiced
- 2 apples, juiced
- 2 oranges, juiced
- 2 c. water (optional)

Directions

Peel apples, oranges, lemons and limes. Using a juicer, juice the basil, limes, lemons, apples and oranges. Pour into glasses, add water if too strong for your taste. Serve with a sprig of basil.

> **Fun Fact**
>
> A single citrus plant can have as many as 60,000 flowers, but only 1 percent of those flowers will turn into fruit.

Snapin Carrot Juice

Preparation: 10 Min.   Makes 2-4 Servings

Ingredients

- 3 large carrots, juiced
- 2 inch piece ginger

Directions

Using a juicer, juice carrots and ginger. Pour into a glass and enjoy.

Hazelnut Drink

Preparation: 10 Min. *Makes 2-4 Servings*

Ingredients

- 2 c. hazelnut milk (page 142)
- 2 tbsp. coconut nectar
- 1 ¾ c. coconut water
- 4 tbsp. shredded unsweetened coconut

Fun Fact

Torches made of hazelnut wood were used during ancient Roman wedding ceremonies because they believed that hazelnut ensured long happy and prosperous marriage

Directions

Soak hazelnuts overnight. Drain off the water and place nuts in a blender and make milk. Save pulp for cookies or other food.

Add coconut nectar, coconut water, unsweetened coconut and water to milk in blender and mix until smooth.

Place a cheesecloth over a bowl and pour blender mix and strain. This will ensure that the drink is smooth.

Garnish with cinnamon and serve. May pour drink over ice just before serving.

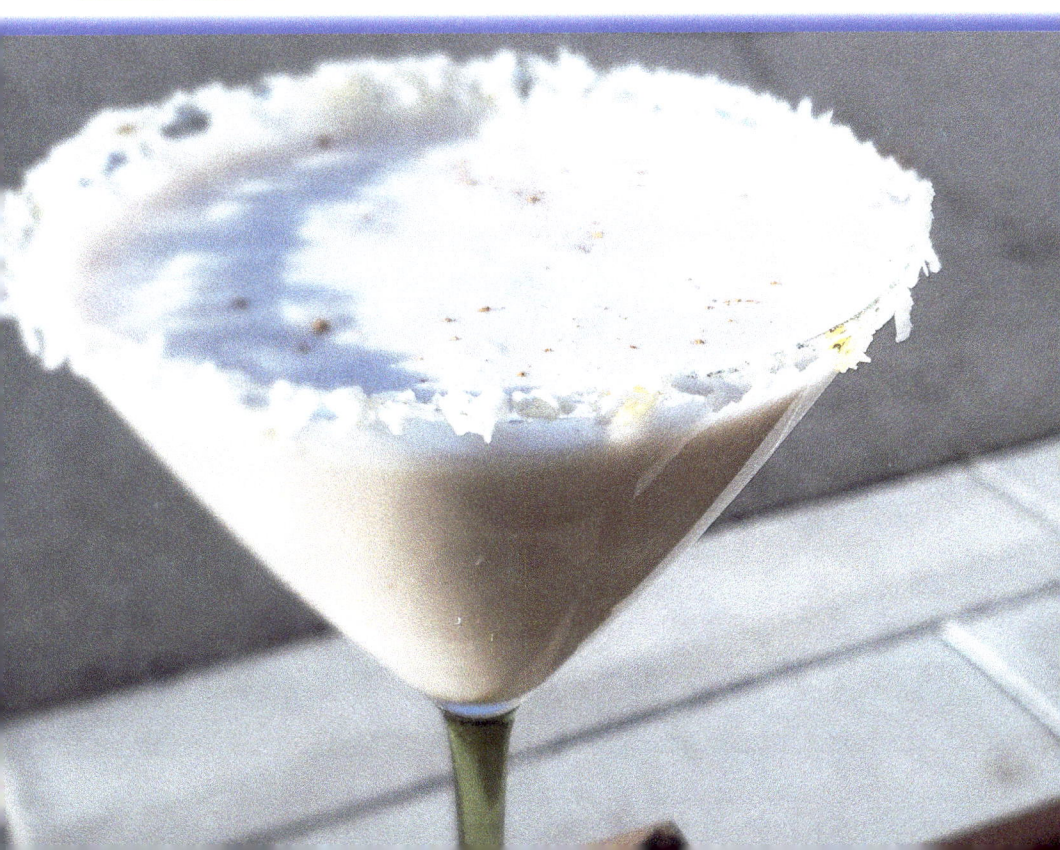

Tabbouleh Smoothie

Preparation: *Makes 2-4*
5 Min. *Servings*

Ingredients

- hemp seed milk (page 142)
- 3 tomatoes
- 1 cucumber
- 2 green onions
- 2 c. fresh parsley
- ½ c. fresh mint
- 1 lemon, juice

Directions

Make hemp seed milk. Peel cucumber and place in blender with tomatoes, green onions, parsley, mint, hemp seed milk, and lemon juice.

Blend until smooth. Serve in a glass with a mint sprig for garnish.

Variation

Other nut or seed milks can be used in place of hemp seed milk

---

Rejuvelac

Preparation: *Sprouting:* *Fermenting:* *Makes 1*
10 Min. *1-3 Days* *2-4 Days* *Gallon*

Ingredients

- 1 c. sprouted wheat, ½ -1 inch tail
- 1 gallon water

Directions

Sprout wheat for one to 3 days. The wheat should have a ½ -1 inch tail.

Drain soaking water and place wheat in a food processor. Add 2 cups of pure water and pulse blender for 2-3 minutes until everything is well blended.

Pour into a gallon picture and add remaining water. Stir the liquid and then cover with cheesecloth.

Stir the liquid 2 to 4 times a day for 2 to 3 days. After fermentation strain wheat from water and refrigerate liquid. You should have a slightly lemony flavor when done. If it stinks really bad, it is no good.

Fun Fact

Rejuvelac is a fermented grain water that was invented by Ann Wigmore.

It is closely related to a traditional Romanian drink, called borș, a fermented wheat bran that can be used to make a sour soup called ciorbă.

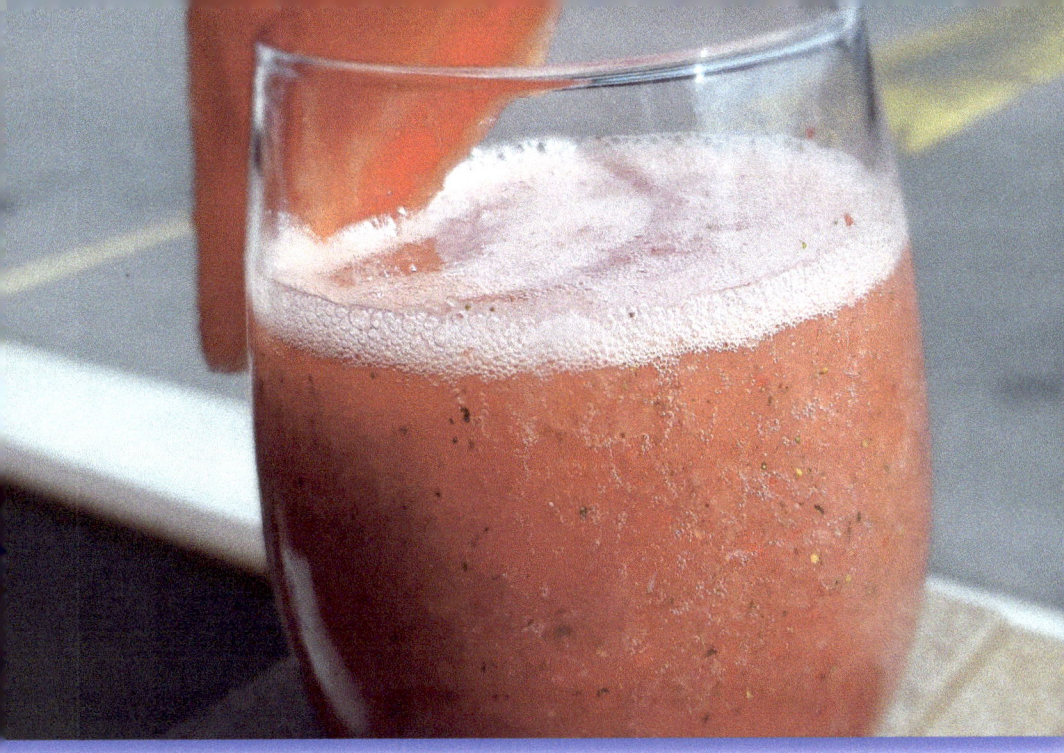

Watermelon Strawberry Drink

Preparation: 10 Min.   Makes 2-4 Servings

Ingredients

- 2 c. strawberries
- 2 c. watermelon
- 1 c. crushed ice
- 1 tbsp. fresh or dried stevia leaves
- 1 c. water (optional)
- fresh mint, for garnish (optional)

Directions

Puree strawberries, watermelon, ice, and stevia until smooth.

Pour into tall glasses and top with water if desired. Garnish with mint and serve.

Fun Facts

Not only does watermelon satisfy thirst and helps with hydration it is a source of electrolytes that help nerve cell communication, muscle contraction and heart functions

If you are in China or Japan a good gift to give the host is watermelon. In Egypt and Israel salty feta cheese is paired with sweet watermelon.

Sweet Summer Soup

Preparation: 25 Min.   Chilling: 2-8 Hrs.   Makes 4-6 Servings

Ingredients

Base

- ½ c. macadamia nuts
- ½ tsp. vanilla
- ½ c. pure water
- 1 orange
- 1 tsp. mint
- ½ tsp. cinnamon, ground

Fruit

- 1 c. strawberries
- 1 c. cantaloupe
- 1 c. orange
- 1 c. pineapple
- 1 c. honeydew

Directions

Place peeled orange in a blender. Add macadamia nuts, vanilla, mint, cinnamon and water, blend until smooth. Chill while preparing fruit.

In a bowl, prepare and place sliced strawberries, chopped cantaloupe, orange, pineapple, and honeydew.
Pour macadamia nut mixture over fruit and gently mix.

Chill at least 2 hours. Garnish with orange segments and mint.

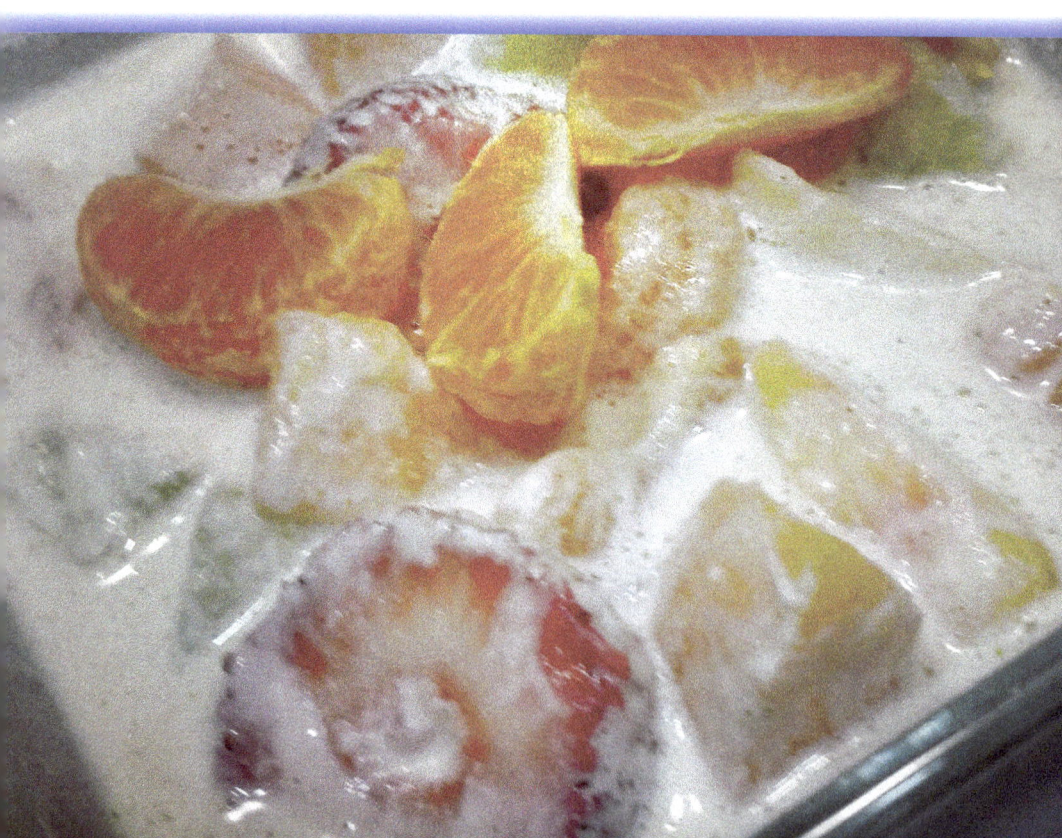

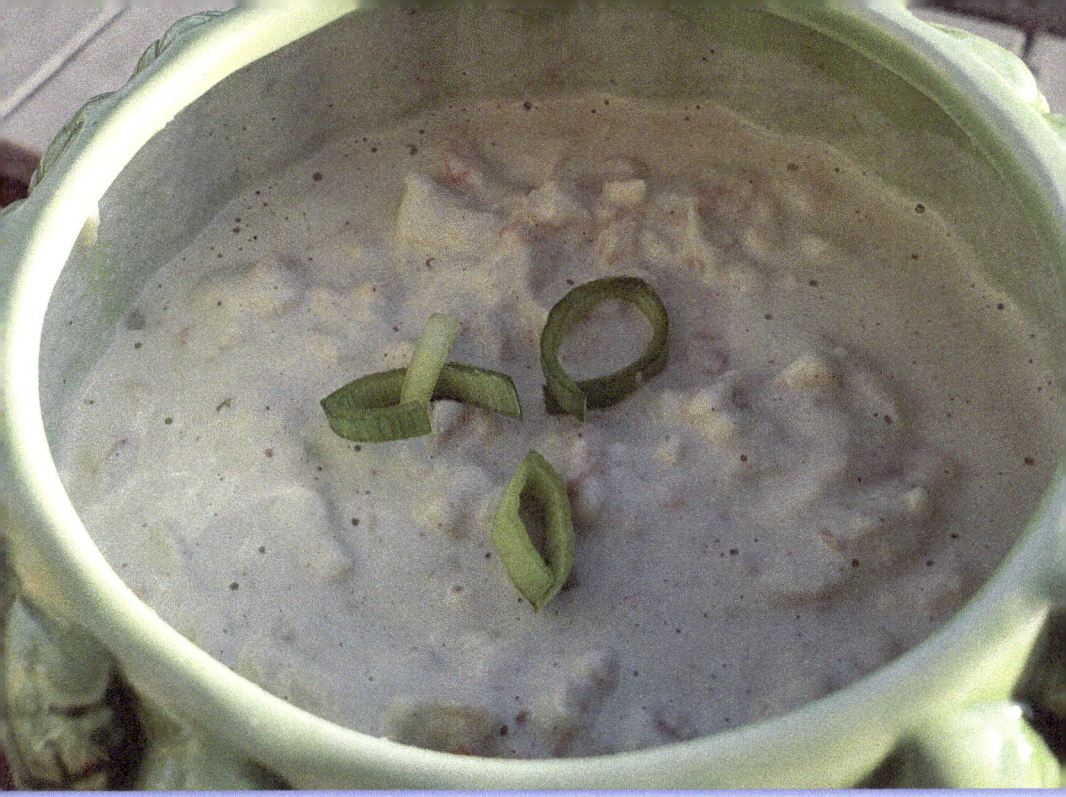

Parsnip Chowder

Preparation: 30 Min.

Makes 4-6 Servings

Ingredients

- 1 c. carrots, diced
- 1 c. jicama, diced
- 2 c. parsnips, diced
- 1 ½ c. onion, diced
- 1 ½ c. water
- ¾ c. cashews
- 1 tsp. Himalayan crystal salt
- ½ tsp. white pepper
- 1 tbsp. cold pressed olive oil
- ½ tsp. turmeric

Directions

Peel and dice parsnips. Dice carrots and jicama then place in a bowl along with parsnips.

In a blender, combine cashews, onion, oil, salt, pepper and turmeric, blend until smooth. If it is too thin, add more cashews.

Pour blender mix over the vegetables and serve.

Fun Fact

Because parsnips store so well above ground as well as underground, parsnips are available year-round. However, the optimal season is fall through spring.

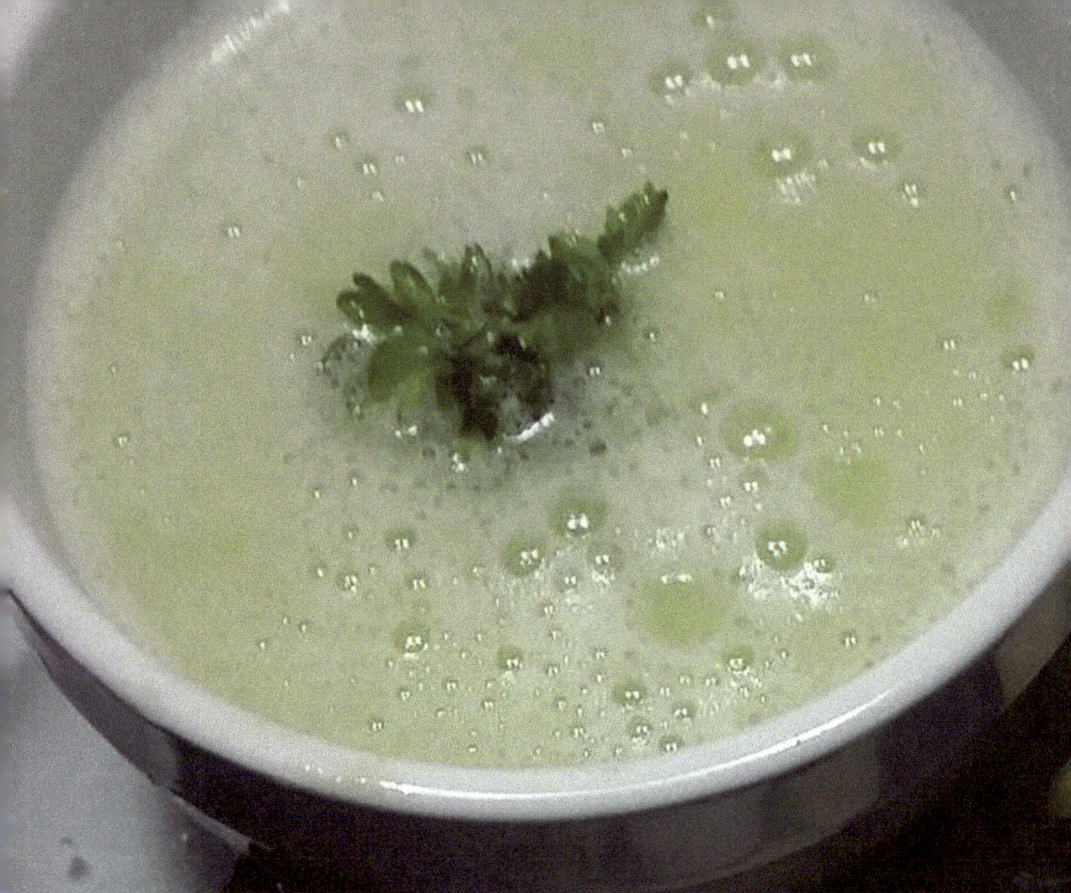

Cool Cucumber Soup

Ingredients

- 2 medium cucumbers
- ½ small onion
- 3 celery stocks, cut into ½ inch pieces
- 1 tbsp. lemon juice or raw apple cider vinegar
- 2 tsp. Himalayan crystal salt
- water as needed
- garnish: parsley

Preparation:
15 Min.

Makes 4-6
Servings

Directions

Blend cucumbers, onion, celery, lemon juice, and salt in a blender until smooth. Adding only enough water to achieve desired.

Garnish the soup with parsley.

Fun Fact

Cool as a cucumber is not just a saying about people but the fact that cucumbers are 20 degrees cooler inside than they are outside.

Pumpkin African Stew

Preparation: 30 Min.
Makes 4-6 Servings

Ingredients

- 2 c. pumpkin
- 1 clove garlic
- 1 ½ c. tomatoes
- 2 green onions
- 1 c. peas
- 1 lemon, juiced
- 1 young coconut
- 1 tsp. chili powder
- 1 tsp. turmeric
- ½ tsp. cumin
- ½ tsp. Himalayan crystal salt
- pepper to taste
- raw pumpkin seeds to garnish

Directions

Peel, seed and cube pumpkin.

In blender, mix young coconut meat and water with 1 cup pumpkin, garlic, green onion, lemon, turmeric, cumin salt, pepper, and chili powder. Blend until smooth and creamy.

In a bowl, place remaining pumpkin, peas, and diced tomatoes. Pour creamy blender mix over the top. Garnish with pumpkin seeds.

Fun Fact

During the Vietnam War pumpkin soup was a staple for the prisoners of war in North Vietnamese prison camps.

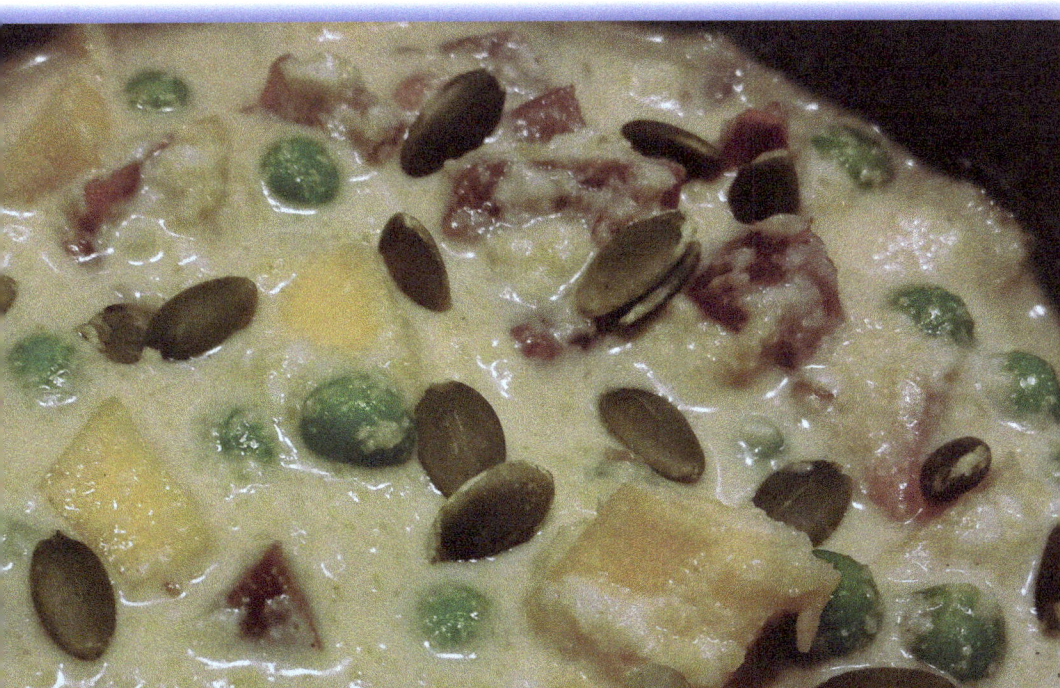

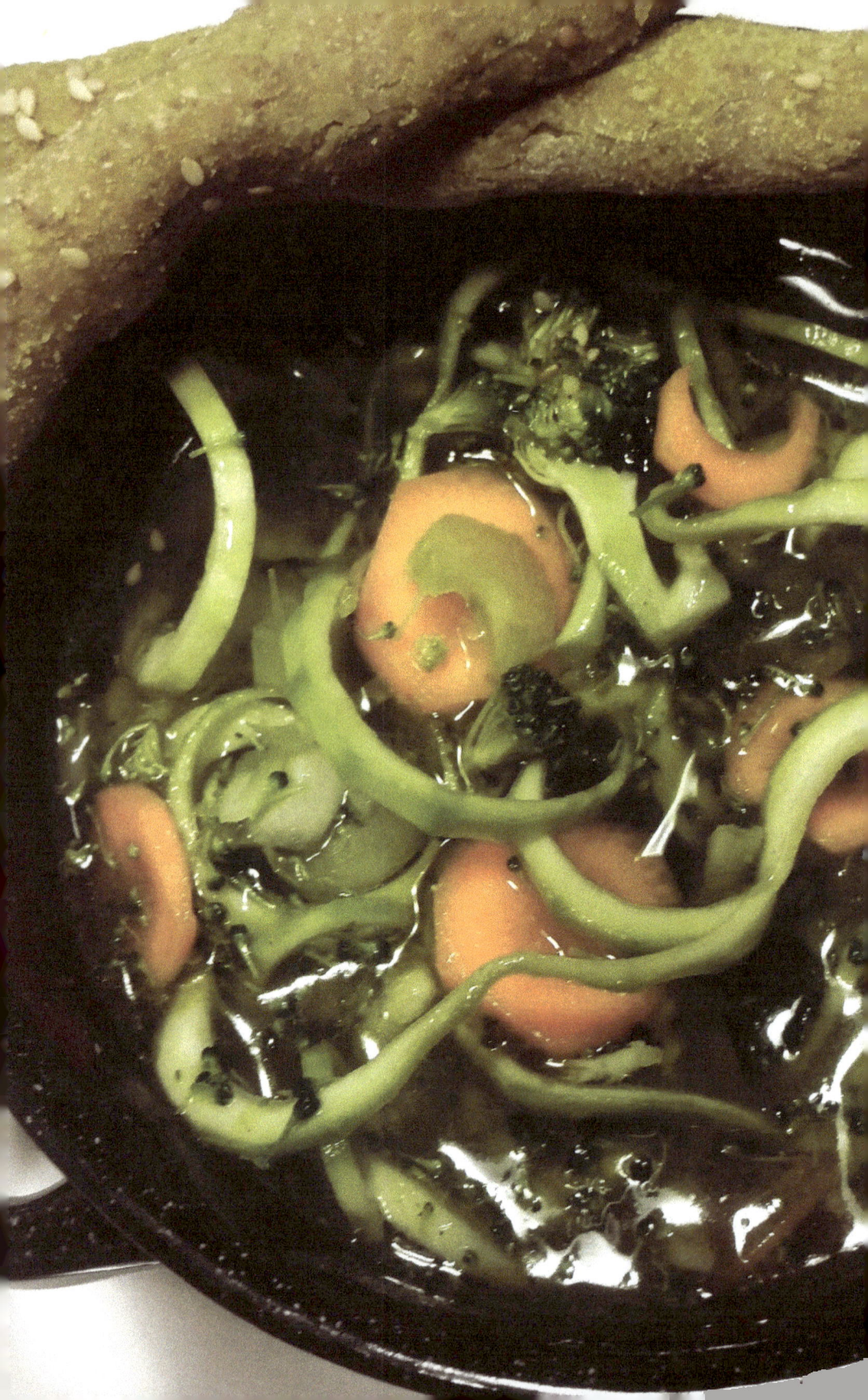

Vegetable "Noodle" Soup

Preparation: 30 Min.   *Makes 4-6 Servings*

Ingredients

Soup Base

- 2 c. pure water
- 2 tsp. cold pressed olive oil
- ½ c. celery
- ½ c. onion
- ¼ tsp. poultry seasoning
- 2 tsp. Himalayan crystal salt
- ½ tsp. white pepper

"Noodles"

- ½ c. celery, sliced
- 1 c. carrot
- 1 c. zucchini
- ½ c. broccoli

Directions

In a blender, combine celery, onion, poultry seasoning, salt, pepper, and oil until smooth. Adding enough water to make it the texture and thickness you desire. Set aside.

Prepare noodles by thinly slicing celery and carrots. Chop broccoli then place in a bowl with celery and carrots. Make zucchini noodles using a spiralizer or shred. Cut zucchini into shorter strips add to the bowl.

Cover ingredients in bowl with blended soup base. Add more salt and pepper if desired.

Vegetable Soup Base

Preparation: 10 Min.   *Makes 2-4 Servings*

Ingredients

- ½ c. onion
- 1 c. turnip
- 1 c. parsnip
- 8 c. celery
- 1 zucchini, diced
- Himalayan crystal salt
- pepper to taste

Note

For winter, use dried vegetables or from root cellar.

Directions

Combine onion, carrots, turnip, parsnip, and celery in a blender.

Pour mixture into milk bag or a clean nylon knee high and strain over a bowl.

Squeeze to make sure all the liquid is out. Add salt and pepper to juice and let set for at least an hour.

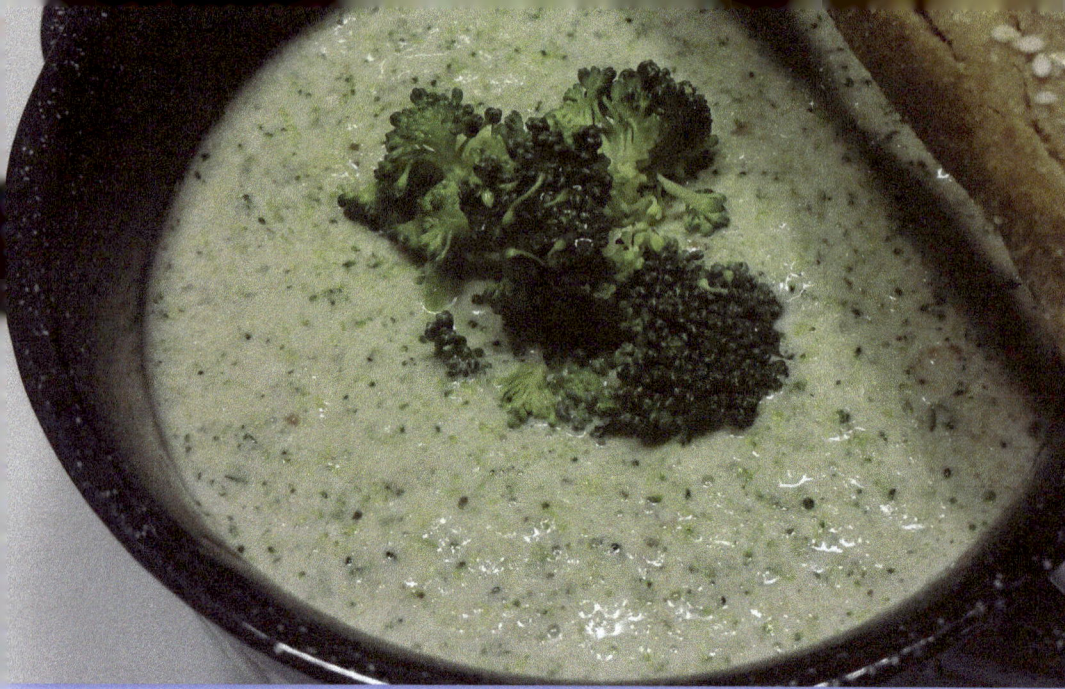

Broccoli Soup

Preparation: 30 Min. *Makes 4-6 Servings*

Ingredients

- 1-2 tsp. cold pressed olive oil
- 1 clove garlic, minced
- ¼ cup onion, minced
- 1 c. cashews
- 2-4 c. water
- 2-4 c. broccoli
- 2 tbsp. parsley
- Himalayan crystal salt to taste
- 1 lemon, juiced
- 2 celery stalks, thinly sliced
- 1 c. cherry tomatoes
- 1 avocado, cubed
- 1 tsp. kelp

Directions

In a blender, purée cashews, onion, garlic, olive oil, broccoli, parsley, and lemon juice add water as needed blend until smooth and the desired consistency is achieved.

I like to have floaters in my soups; there are many different kinds for this soup. You can cube and cut celery, avocado, or broccoli floweret.

Pour purée into a bowl and place the floaters on top just before serving.

Fun Fact

Cup for cup, broccoli has as much vitamin C as an orange, almost as much calcium as milk, and the same amount of protein as a cup of rice.

Mexican Vegetable Soup

Preparation: 30 Min. *Drying:* 30 -90 Min. *Makes 4-6 Servings*

Ingredients

- 1 tbsp. cold pressed olive oil
- ½ yellow or orange bell pepper, diced
- 1 red bell pepper, diced
- 1 tbsp. ground cumin
- ½ tsp. dried oregano
- ¼ tsp. cayenne pepper
- 1 tomatoes, diced
- 1 tbsp. jalapeno pepper, diced
- 2 c. vegetable soup base (page 31)
- 1 c. corn kernels
- 1 zucchini, diced
- Himalayan crystal salt
- pepper to taste

Optional Toppings

- lime juice
- avocado
- cilantro
- sour cream (page 144)

Directions

Make vegetable base and set aside. In a bowl, place bell peppers, jalapeno, zucchini, corn, salt, cumin, oregano, cayenne pepper, and pepper.

Pour vegetable base over vegetable and stir. Place in dehydrator for about 1-3 hours to warm if desired. Add tomatoes and any optional toppings. Serve immediately.

Fun Fact

Americans eat more than 10 billion bowls of soup each year.

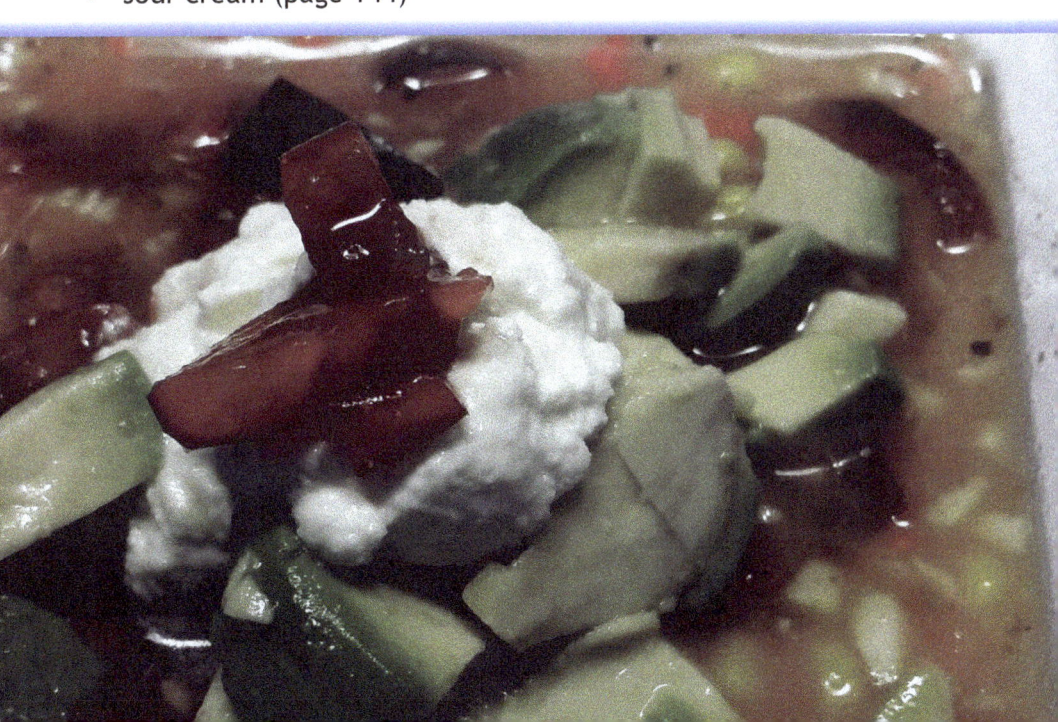

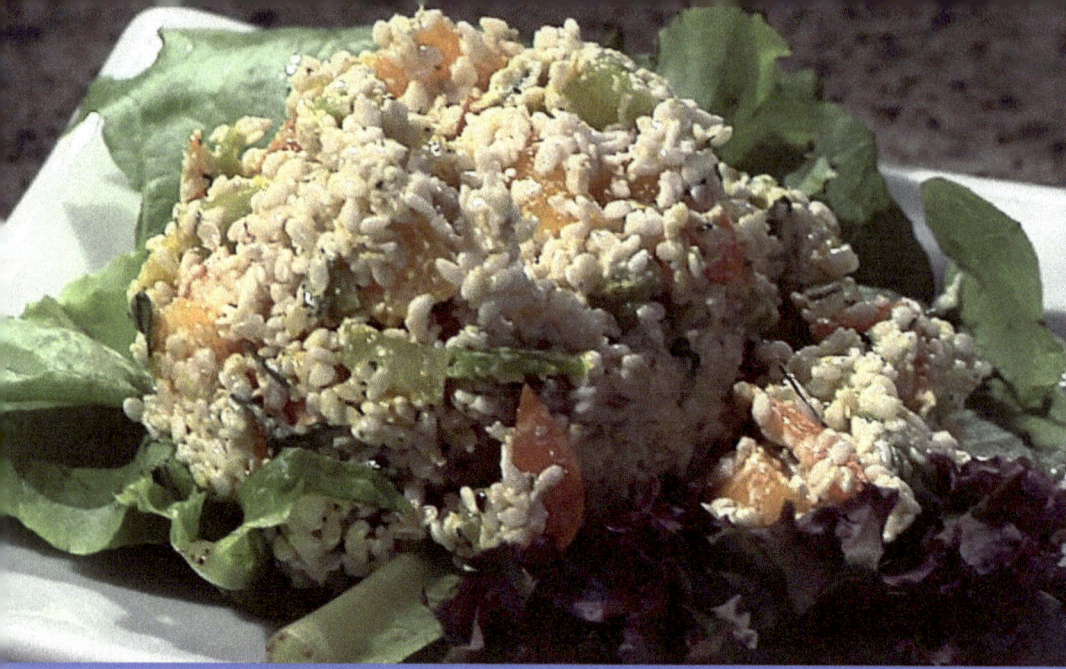

Eggless Salad

Ingredients

- 2 c. sesame seed pulp, from making milk
- 1 red bell pepper, chopped
- 1 small celery, sliced
- 2 green onions, chopped
- 1 tbsp. parsley
- 1 tbsp. dill
- 1 tsp. mustard seed powder
- 1 tbsp. turmeric
- 2 tsp. lovage
- ¼ c. nut mayo (page 143)

Preparation: 30 Min.

Makes 4-6 Servings

Directions

Place sesame seed pulp saved from making sesame milk in a bowl. Chop bell peppers, green onions, parsley, and shredded carrots place in a bowl with sesame pulp.

Add dill, mustard seeds powder, turmeric, lovage and nut mayo mix well. Adjust seasonings to taste. Enjoy as a refreshing salad or stuff it in a tomato or bell pepper.

Fun Fact

Lovage may be a relatively unknown perennial herb today, but it was well-known to the ancient Greeks and Romans who used it as both a culinary and medicinal herb. In Europe, it is known as the Maggi plant.

Smart Cat Salad

Preparation: 25 Min.   Sprouting: 3-5 days   Makes 6-8 Servings

Ingredients

- 1 c. garbanzo beans
- 1 c. cucumber
- ¼ c. red onion
- 1 c. cherry tomatoes
- ½ c. broccoli
- 3 c. lettuce
- ½ c. cauliflower
- ½ c. radish
- 1 bell pepper, red or range
- sprouts
- creamy lemon poppy seed dressing (page 51)

Directions

Sprout garbanzo beans, they should be soft and easily smashed with a fork.

Wash lettuce and place in a bowl or on a plate. Slice cucumber, onion, radish and bell pepper arrange on top of the lettuce. Cut cauliflower and broccoli into small pieces and sprinkle over the salad along with cherry tomatoes and garbanzo beans.

Make the lemon poppy seed dressing and pour over the top of the salad.

How to sprout garbanzo beans

Soak garbanzo beans overnight. Drain and rinse them thoroughly. Invert jar over a bowl at an angle so that the beans will drain and still allow air to circulate. Repeat rinsing and draining 2-3 times per day until sprouts are the desired length, usually 3-6 days.

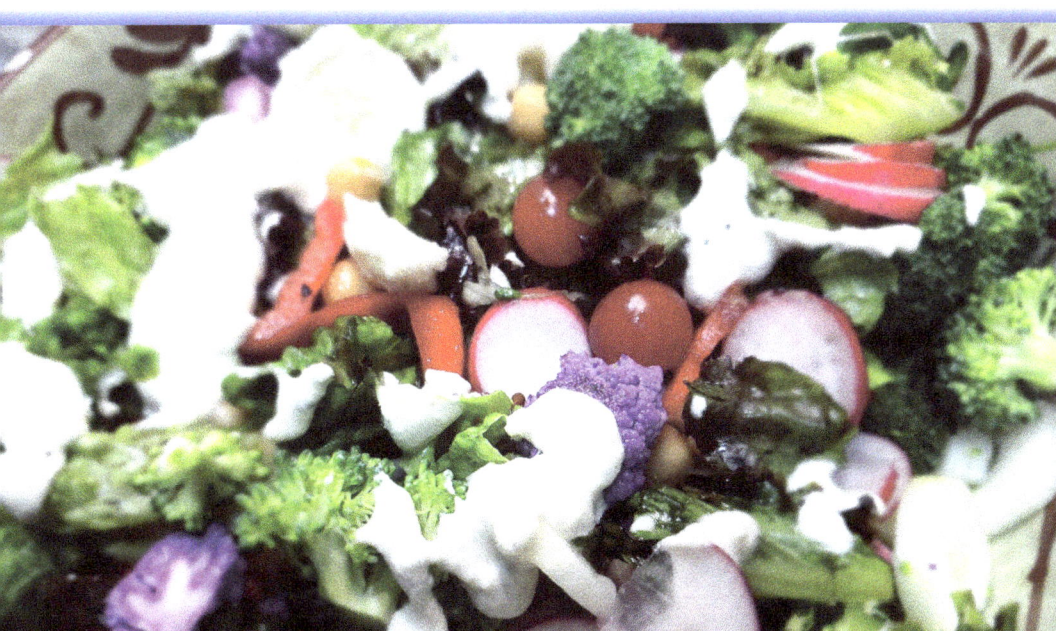

Falafel Salad

Preparation: 15 Min. *Makes 4-6 Servings*

Ingredients

- falafel patties (page 37)

Tahini Dressing

- ¾ c. raw tahini
- 1 lemon juiced
- ¼ c. parsley
- 1 garlic clove
- ½ tsp. paprika
- ½ tsp. Himalayan crystal salt
- ½ tsp. pepper
- Water as needed to thin

Salad

- 3 c. cabbage, shredded
- 3 carrots, shredded
- ¼ c. red onion, thinly sliced

Directions

Make falafel patties and set aside.

Dressing:

In a blender, combine tahini, lemon juice, parsley, paprika salt and pepper. Add water as needed to achieve desired thickness.

Salad:

Wash and shred cabbage and carrots and place in a bowl or on a plate. Thinly slice red onion and toss with cabbage.

Place falafel patties on top of cabbage and pour tahini dressing over top just before serving.

Fun Fact

Falafel has been considered a national dish of Egypt, Palestine, and Israel.

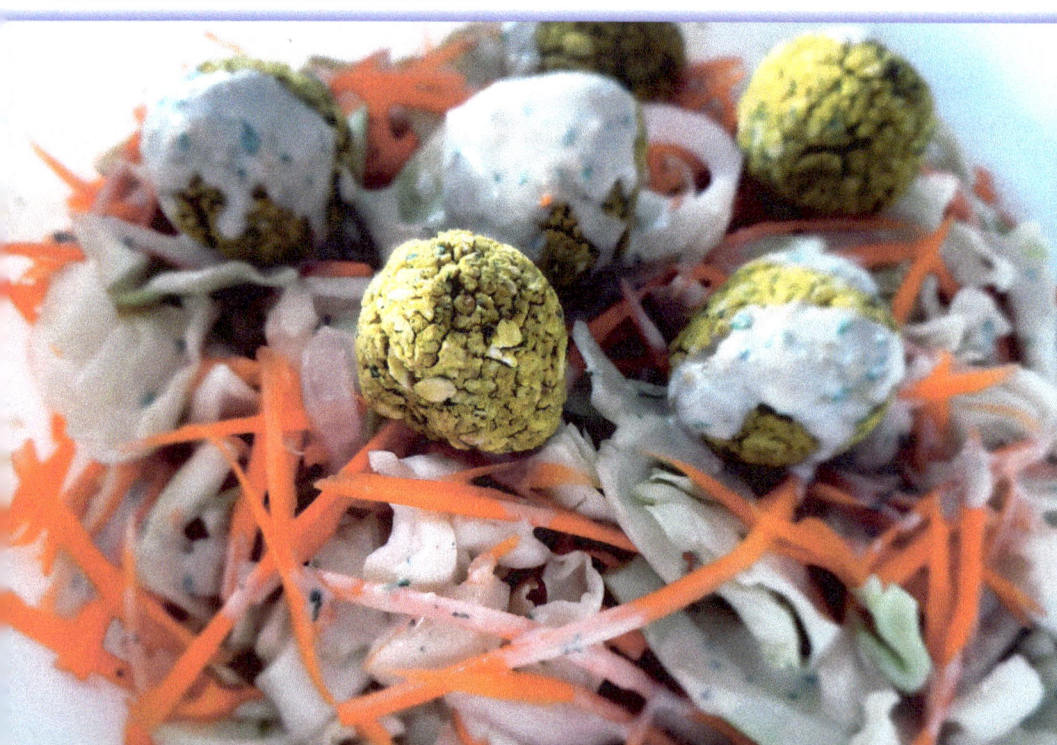

Falafel Patties (balls)

Preparation: 20 Min. *Soaking:* 8-12 Hrs. *Drying:* 2-4 Hrs. *Makes 4-6 Servings*

Ingredients

- 2 c. garbanzo beans
- ½ c. oat groats
- 1-2 cloves garlic
- 2 tbsp. poultry seasoning
- Himalayan crystal salt
- black pepper to taste
- 2 tbsp. water
- 1 tsp. cold pressed olive oil
- 1 tsp. turmeric
- 1 tsp. lemon juice
- handful of fresh parsley

Directions

Sprout garbanzo beans (see page 35). Grind oat groats in a coffee grinder then place in food processor. To food processor, add garbanzo beans, garlic, seasoning, olive oil, lemon juice and parsley. Blend ingredients until smooth, adding water if needed.

Shape mixture into patties about ½ inch thick. Place on nonstick dehydrator sheet and dry 1-2 hours at 100° F. Turn patties and continue drying another hour or until the patties reach the desired dryness.

Fun Fact

The first instance of frying dough made from beans was recorded as a meal in Medieval Egypt, where it was enjoyed by Copts, a Christian ethnic group ate a mainly vegan diet.

Carrot Raisin Salad

Preparation: 15 Min. *Makes 4-6 Servings*

Ingredients

- 1 c. raisins
- 2 apples, shredded
- 3 large carrots, shredded
- ½ c. nut mayo (page 143)
- Himalayan crystal salt

Note

If raisins are hard, soak for 10 minutes to soften then drain off water.

Directions

Shred carrots and apples and place in a medium bowl, add raisins.

Gently mix in the nut mayonnaise and salt. Chill a few hours before serving.

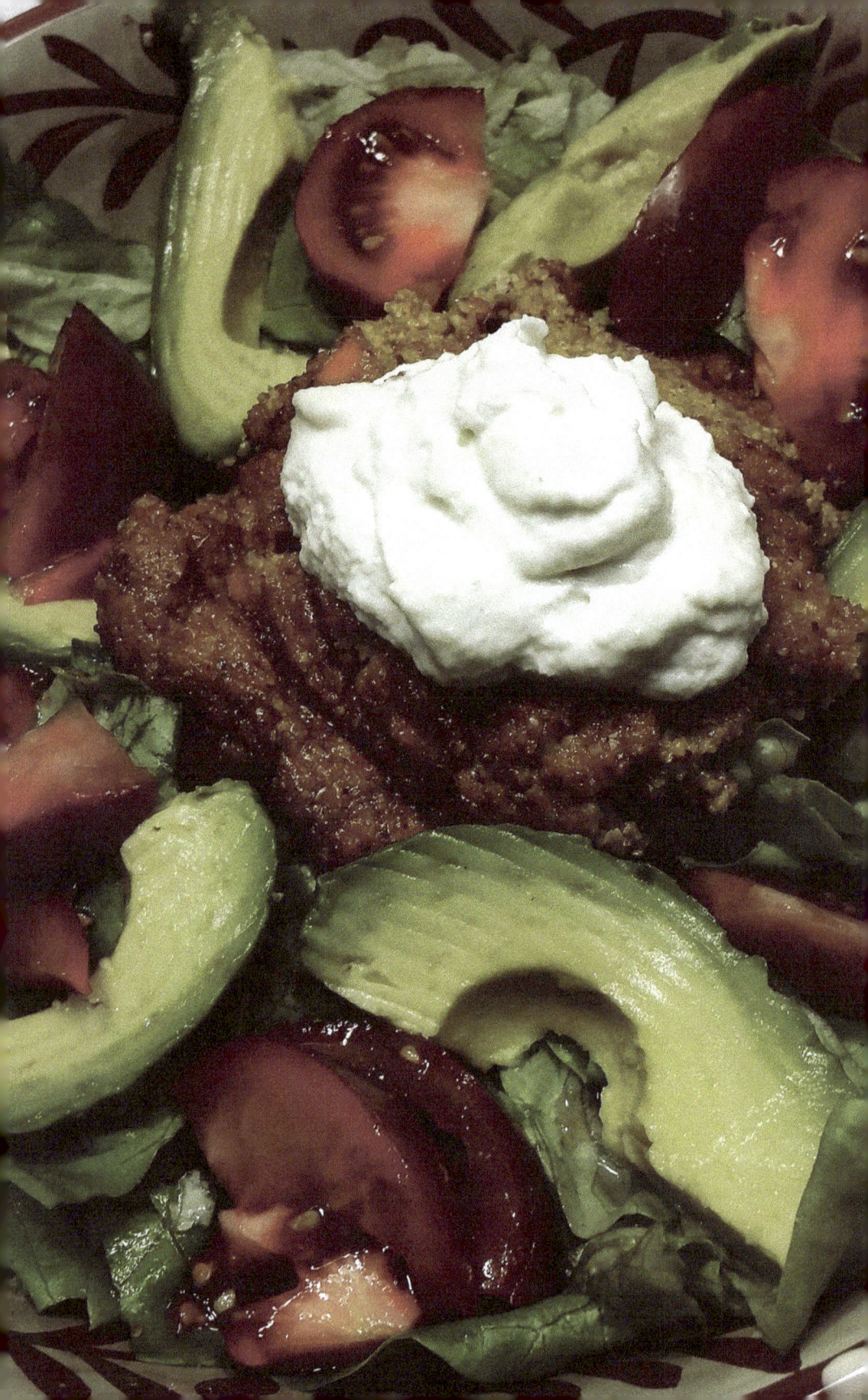

Taco Salad

Preparation: 20 Min. *Makes 4-6 Servings*

Ingredients

- 1 head lettuce, torn into bite sized pieces.
- 2 avocados, sliced
- 4 tomatoes, sliced
- salsa (page 59)
- sour cream (page 144)
- sunflower beans (page 56)
- sundried olives (optional)

Directions

Make sunflower beans and set aside. Wash lettuce, tear into bite sized pieces and place on a plate.

Place a scoopful of sunflower beans onto center of plate on top of the lettuce. Make salsa and place on top of beans.

Arrange tomato, avocado slices, and olive round beans. Drizzle sour cream over the top.

Fun Fact

Dried olives are made by washing then laying them out on trays, and drying them at a low temperature. They are then marinated in olive oil with or without spices.

Fiesta Salad

Preparation: 10 Min. *Makes 2-4 Servings*

Ingredients

- 3 c. spring mix
- 3 c. favorite lettuce
- 1 avocado, cubed
- 1 c. cherry tomatoes
- ½ c. sundried olives
- lime slices, garnish
- 5 artichoke hearts, frozen or water packed (optional not a raw product)
- ½ c. vegan basil feta cheese (page 149, optional)

Fiesta Dressing

- 2 tbsp. cold pressed olive oil
- 1 green onion, chopped
- 1 lime, juiced
- Himalayan crystal salt to taste
- white pepper to taste

Directions

In a small bowl, mix the dressing by hand and set aside. Prepare and place the salad ingredients, except for the avocados, In a large bowl.

Pour Fiesta Dressing over and let mingle about 30 minutes. Add avocado and feta just before serving. Garnish with lime slices.

Fun Fact

Avocados are an Aztec symbol of love and fertility, as they grow in pairs on trees.

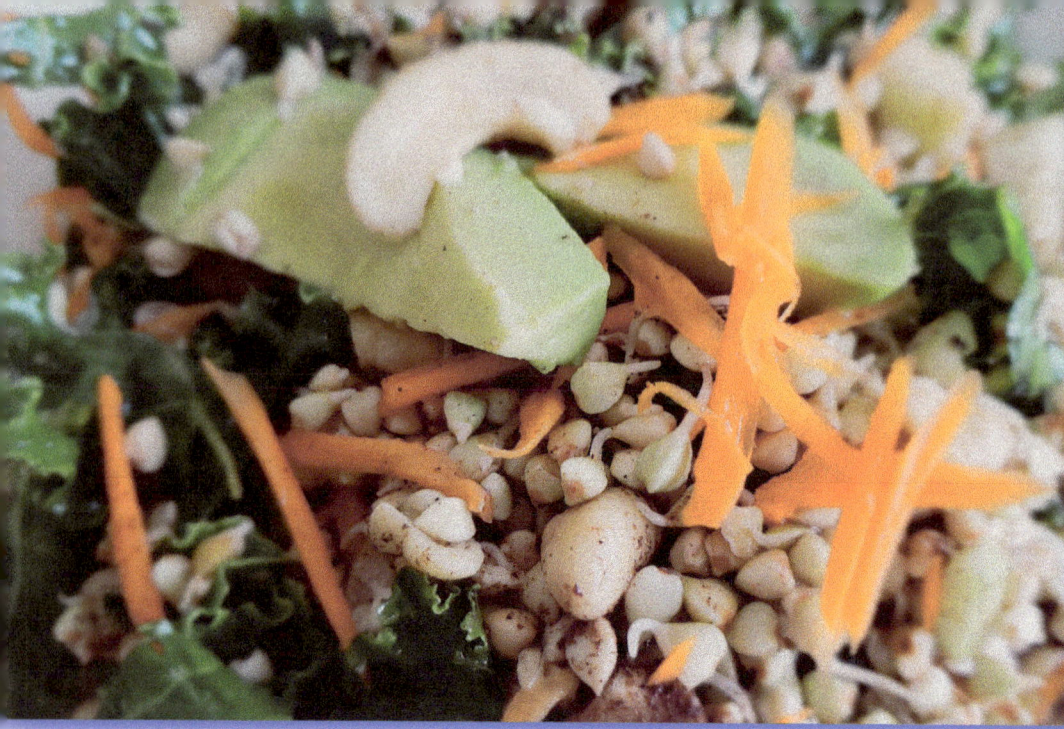

Moroccan Buckwheat Salad

Preparation: 10 Min.   Chilling: 1-2 Hrs.   Makes 4-6 Servings

Ingredients

- 1 c. buckwheat groats, soaked
- handful kale
- ½ c. carrots
- 1 avocado
- 1 lemon, juiced
- 1 c. zucchini, chopped
- ½ c. cashews (optional)
- 1 tsp. cinnamon
- 1 tsp. allspice
- ¼ c. fresh mint, chopped
- ½ tsp. Himalayan crystal salt
- pepper to taste
- 1 tsp. cold pressed olive oil

Directions

Soak buckwheat overnight. Drain off water and rinse then place buckwheat into a bowl.

Wash kale, remove the steam, tear kale into small pieces, and add to the bowl with buckwheat.

Chop mint, shred carrots, slice zucchini and cube avocados them toss them in with the buckwheat and kale then mix in cashews.

Place lemon juice in a small bowl with olive oil, cinnamon, allspice, salt and pepper mix, toss salad with dressing.

Fun Fact

Buckwheat is a relative of rhubarb.

Old Fashioned "Potato" Salad

Preparation: 20 Min.
Makes 4-6 Servings

Ingredients

- 1 large jicama, peeled and cubed
- 3 stocks celery, sliced
- 2 green onions, chopped
- 2 medium cucumbers, sliced
- 1 small red, yellow, or orange bell pepper
- 6 radishes
- ½ tsp. raw apple cider vinegar
- 1 ½ tsp. mustard powder
- 1 tbsp. dill
- 1 ½ c. nut mayo (page 143)
- Himalayan crystal salt to taste
- black pepper to taste

Directions

Make nut mayo and place in a bowl. Mix dill, mustard powder, vinegar, salt, and pepper into nut mayo.

Peel and cube jicama, make sure cubes are small and bite sized. Place jicama in a bowl and mix with nut mayo.

Thinly slice celery, cucumbers, bell pepper, radishes and chop green onions. Mix with jicama then refrigerate and serve.

Note

Choose jicama that is firm has few spots and no kicks or broken skin. A nice smooth tan color is desirable. As jicama ages it will wrinkle, dry out and spots will darken.

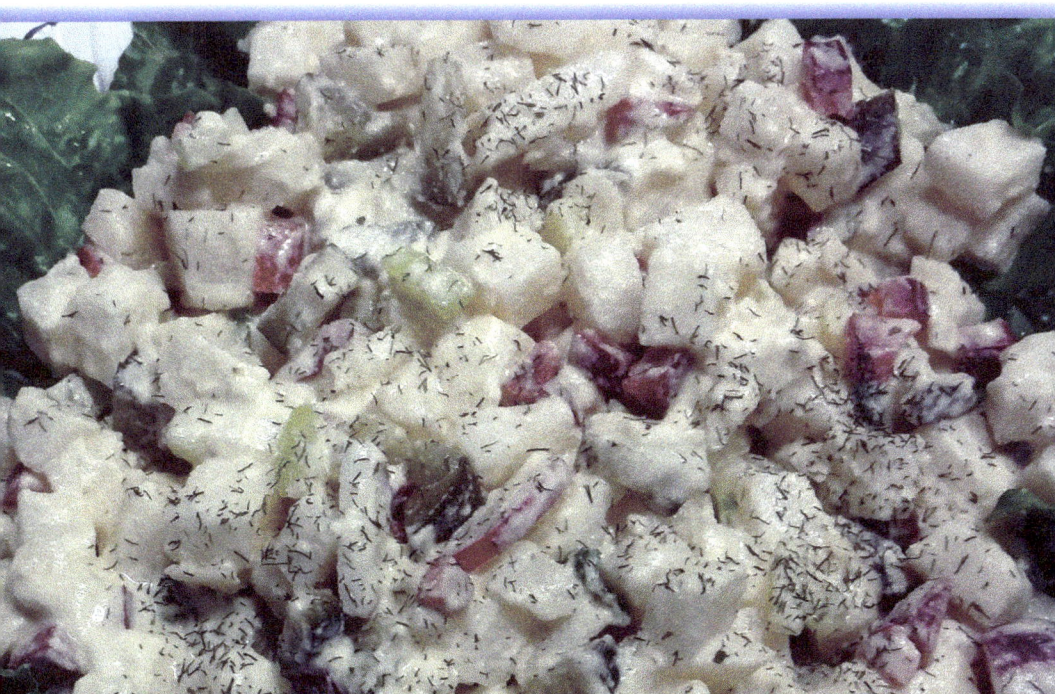

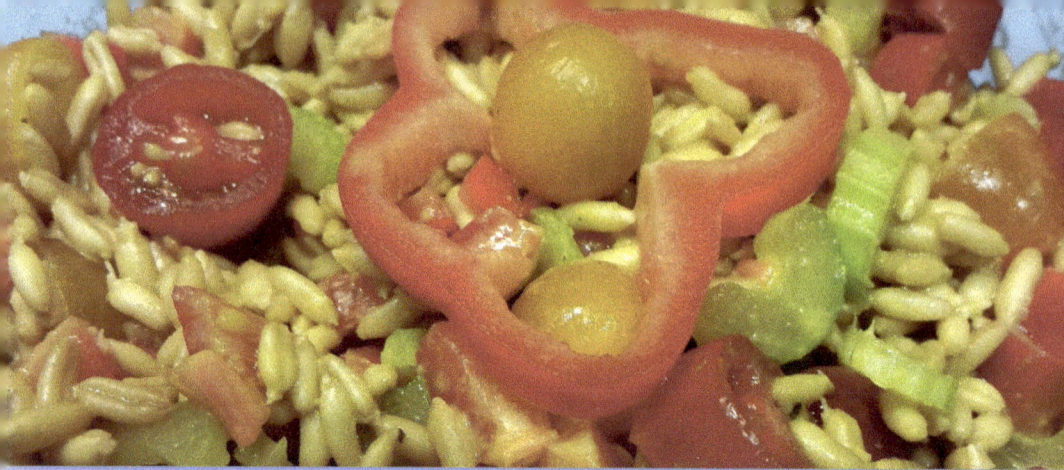

Sprouted Kamut Salad with Vinaigrette

Preparation: 20 Min. *Sprouting:* 2-3 Days *Makes 4-6 Servings*

Ingredients

Salad

- 1 c. kamut or wheat berries, soaked 2 days
- ¾ c. red bell pepper
- ¾ c. yellow bell pepper
- ¾ c. small summer squash
- ¾ c. tomatoes

Vinaigrette

- 3 tbsp. cold pressed olive oil
- 3 tbsp. raw apple cider vinegar
- 2 tbsp. onion powder
- 1 tbsp. pure water
- 1 tbsp. mustard powder
- 1 tbsp. garlic powder
- 1 tsp. cayenne pepper
- 1 tsp. thyme
- ½ tsp. Himalayan crystal salt
- black pepper to taste

Directions

Sprout Kamut (wheat) for about 2 days or until soft.

In a small bowl, mix vinegar, olive oil, onion powder, water, mustard powder, garlic powder, cayenne pepper, thyme, salt, and pepper with a fork or spoon until well mixed.

Cut red and yellow bell peppers into strips, slice squash and chop tomatoes then place in a bowl. Add sprouted Kamut and toss together. Pour vinaigrette over salad and chill at least 3 hours.

Fun Fact

Kamut has a rich, buttery flavor and may be appropriate for individuals with slight wheat sensitivity since it has a low gluten content.

Kale Strawberry Salad

Preparation: 25 Min.   Sprouting: 3-5 days   Makes 6-8 Servings

Ingredients

- 2-3 c. strawberries, halved
- 1 bunch kale
- 1 c. pecans
- ¼ c. basil
- 1 tsp. cold pressed olive oil
- strawberry dressing (page 51, optional)

Directions

Wash kale and remove thick stem. Massage, or rub, in olive oil into each leaf. Tear kale into bite sized pieces and place them in the bowl.

Slice strawberries and chop basil. Toss kale, strawberries and basil together.

Place salad on a plate and top with pecans that have been soaked and dried. May dress with strawberry dressing.

Fun Fact

Belgium has a museum dedicated to strawberries. In the gift shop you can buy everything from strawberry jam to strawberry beer.

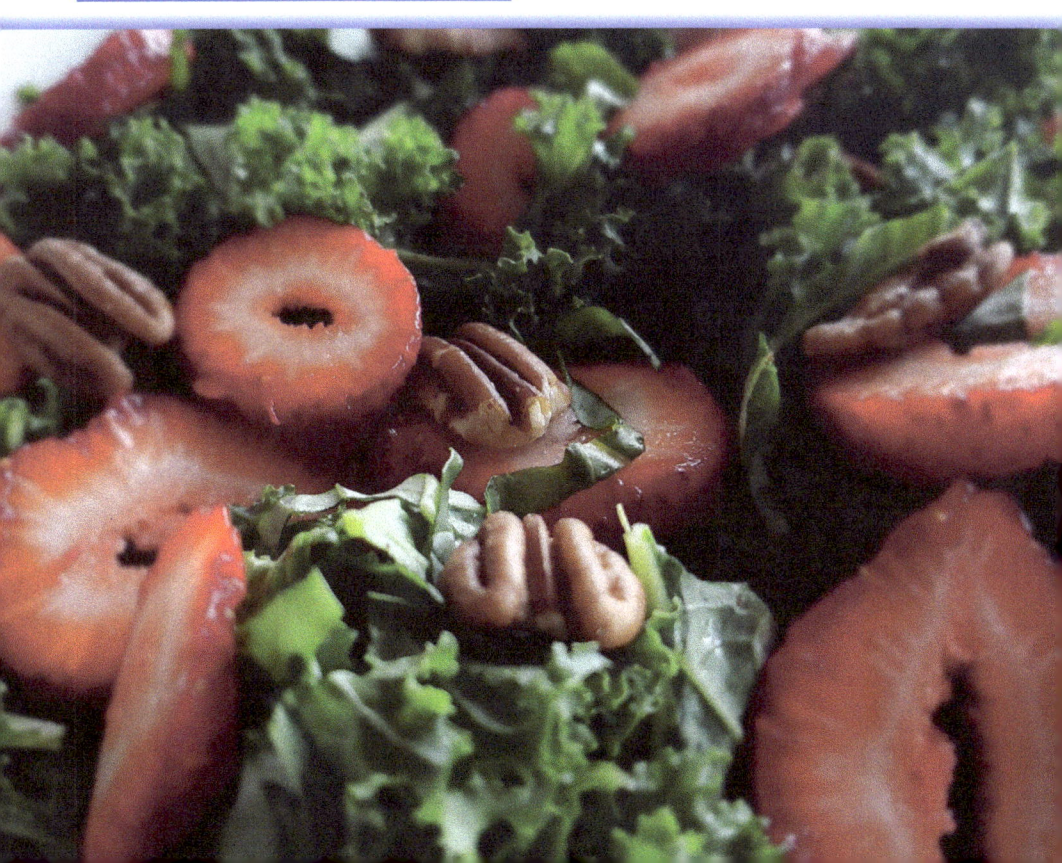

Flora's Albanian Salad

Preparation: 10 Min. *Makes 2-4 Servings*

Ingredients

- 3 cucumbers, sliced
- 1 yellow squash, thinly sliced
- 2 tomatoes, sliced
- ½ red bell pepper
- ½ orange, or yellow bell pepper
- 4 tbsp. cold pressed olive oil
- 3 tbsp. raw apple cider vinegar
- Himalayan crystal salt
- black pepper to taste

Directions

Slice cucumbers, yellow squash, tomatoes, red, orange, and yellow bell pepper then place into a bowl.

In a small jar with a lid, place oil, vinegar, salt, and pepper. Put lid on jar and shake until well mixed.

Pour dressing over vegetables and toss. Arrange on a plate and serve.

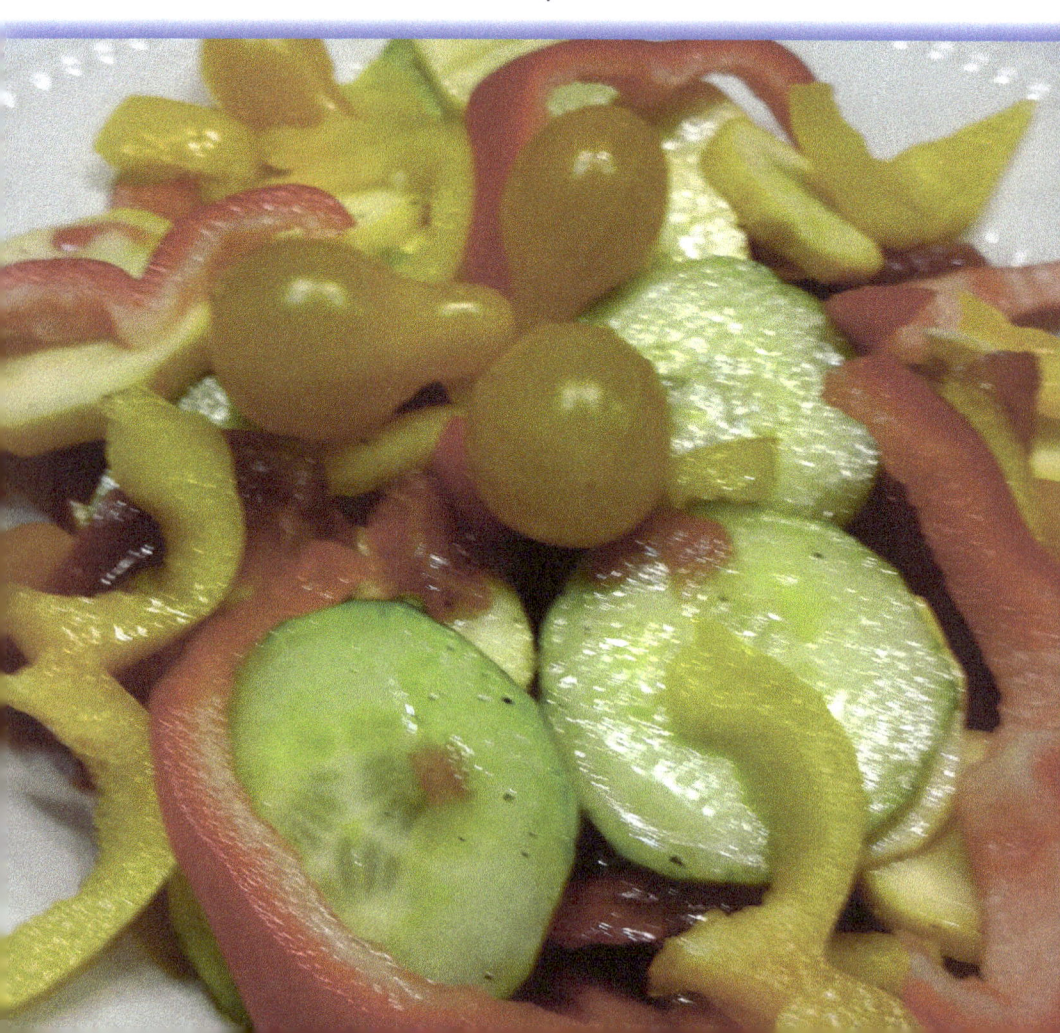

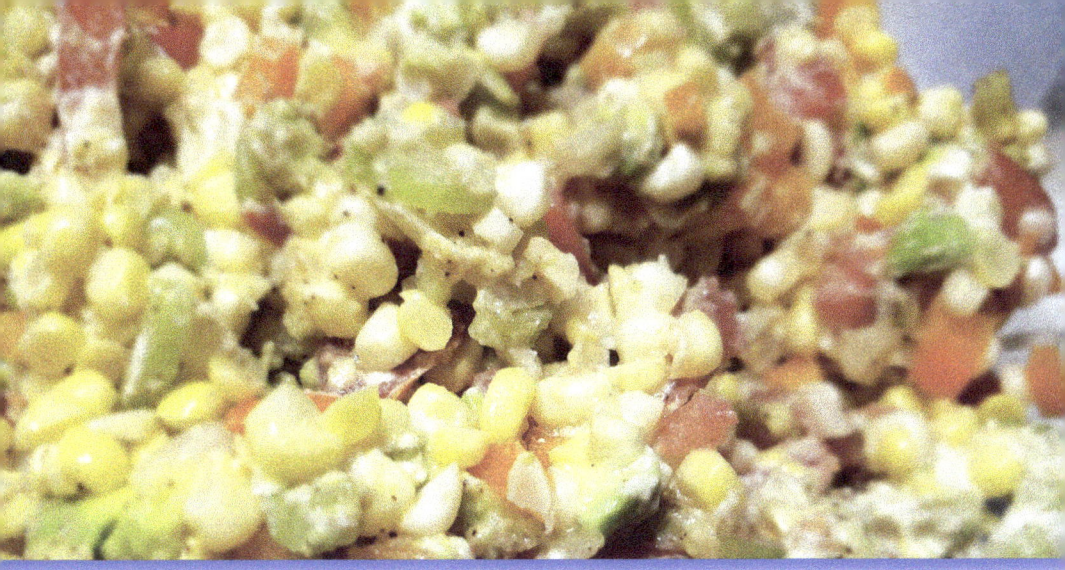

Scrambled Corn Salad

Preparation: 10 Min.

Makes 2-4 Servings

Ingredients

- 2 c. corn kernels
- 1-2 tbsp. cold pressed olive oil
- 1 c. tomato, chopped
- ½ c. celery, chopped
- 1 red bell pepper, minced
- ½ c. onion, minced
- ½ tsp. cumin
- ¾ tsp. turmeric
- ½ tsp. cayenne pepper or black pepper
- 1 avocado, cubed
- ½ c. sour cream (page 144)

Directions

Cut kernels from corn, you may use frozen that have been thawed. In a bowl, combine corn, olive oil, chopped tomato, celery, bell pepper, onion, and spice.

Gently toss together and add cubed avocado. Fold in the almond sour cream and enjoy. May warm to 100°F, before adding almond sour cream, if desired.

Fun Fact

The corn plant is actually a grass, and the kernels are grains, like wheat or oats.

The word "corn" denotes whatever grain is the most popular in an area; for instance, in England, corn refers to wheat, but in Scotland and Ireland, corn is oats and in Germany, corn means rye.

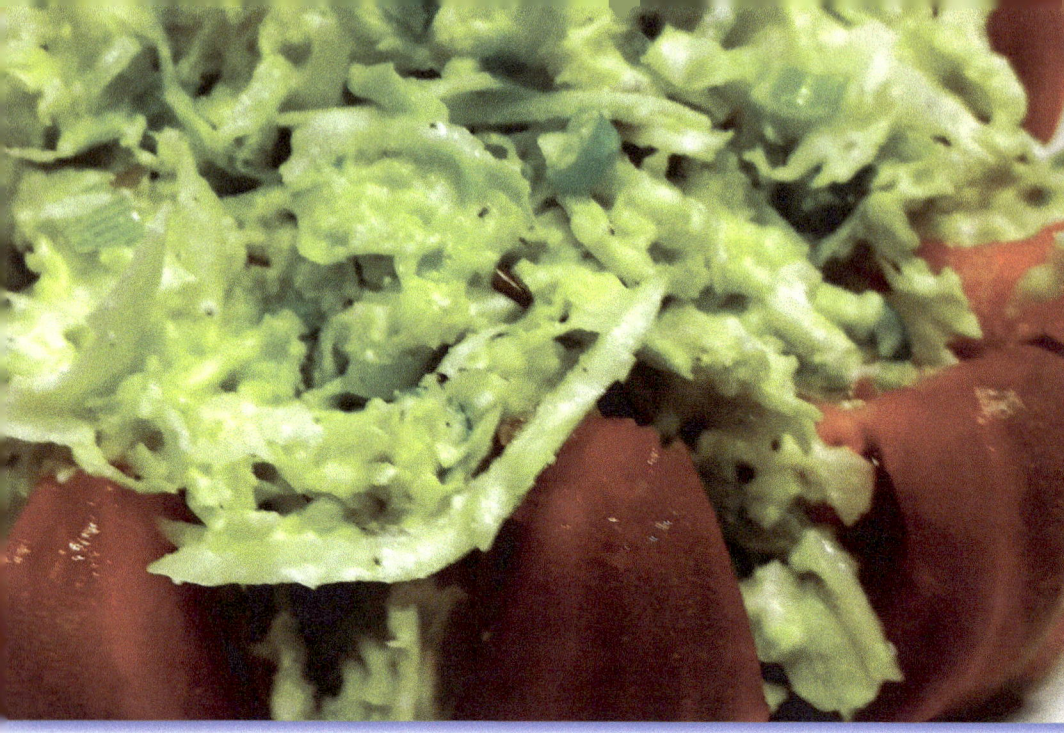

Stuffed Tomato with Cabbage Salad

Preparation: 10 Min. Chilling: 1-2 Hrs. Makes 4-6 Servings

Ingredients

- 2-4 ripe tomatoes
- 1 clove garlic
- 3 c. savoy cabbage
- 1 green onion
- ½ tsp. Himalayan crystal salt
- black pepper to taste
- ¼ c. nut mayo

Directions

Make mayo (page 143) and set aside.

Wash and slice tomatoes, leaving the bottom connected and set aside. It should kind of look like a flower.

Wash and shred cabbage using a mandolin, place in a bowl.

Mince garlic and thinly slice green onion add to cabbage. Mix in garlic and green onion salt and pepper. Gently mix in nut mayo.

Place cabbage salad in the middle of the cut tomato and serve.

> **Fun Fact**
>
> Savoy cabbage is similar to ordinary cabbage, but with a milder flavor the leaves are crunchy, succulent and tender. Savoy is distinguished by its heavily textured, crinkled leaves.

Mediterranean Buckwheat Salad

Preparation: 25 Min. Soaking 8-12 Hrs. Makes 2-4 Servings

Ingredients

Salad

- 1 bell pepper, yellow or orange, diced
- 1 c. cherry tomatoes
- 1 c. cucumber, diced
- ¼ c. parsley, fresh
- ½ c. red onion, diced
- 1 c. buckwheat groats, soaked
- ½ c. dried olives (optional)
- 1 avocado, diced (optional)
- ½ c. vegan feta cheese (page 149)

Dressing

- 4 tsp. cold pressed olive oil
- 1 tsp. oregano, dried
- 1 lemon, juiced
- ¼ tsp. Himalayan crystal salt

Directions

Make vegan feta cheese, using oregano in place of basil.

Soak buckwheat groats overnight. Drain off water and rinse then place in a bowl.

Dice bell pepper, cucumber and red onion and mix with buckwheat, add parsley, cherry tomatoes, olives and avocado gently mix.

Juice lemon then add oil, oregano, and salt then toss with buckwheat salad.

Crumble feta cheese over top just before serving.

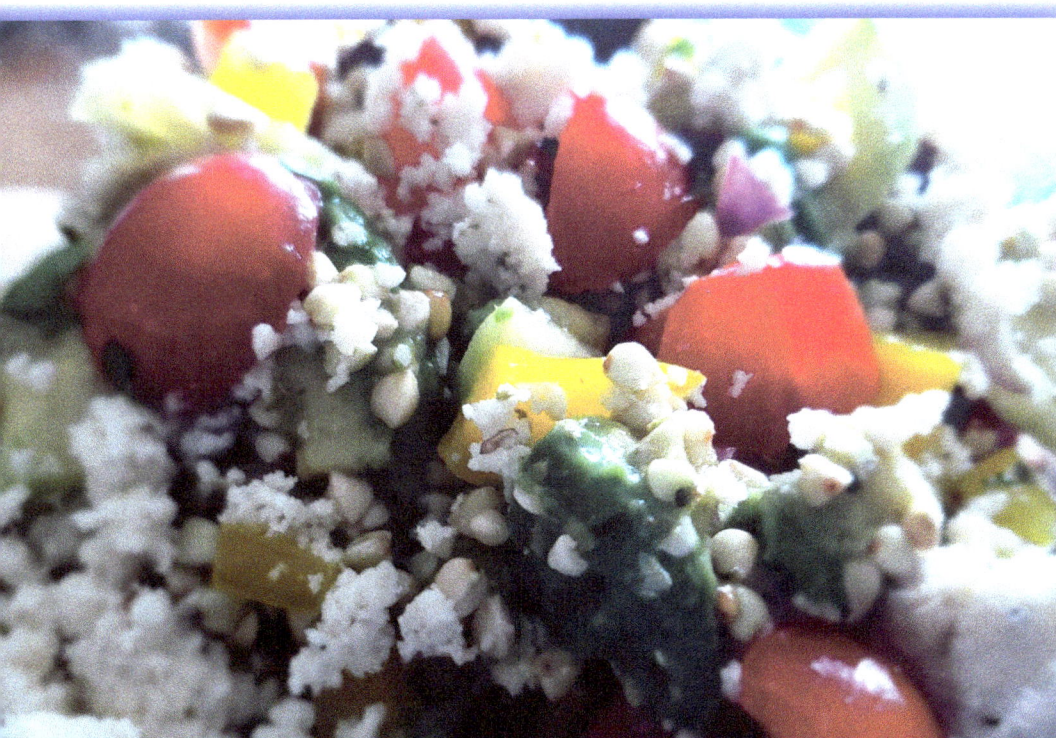

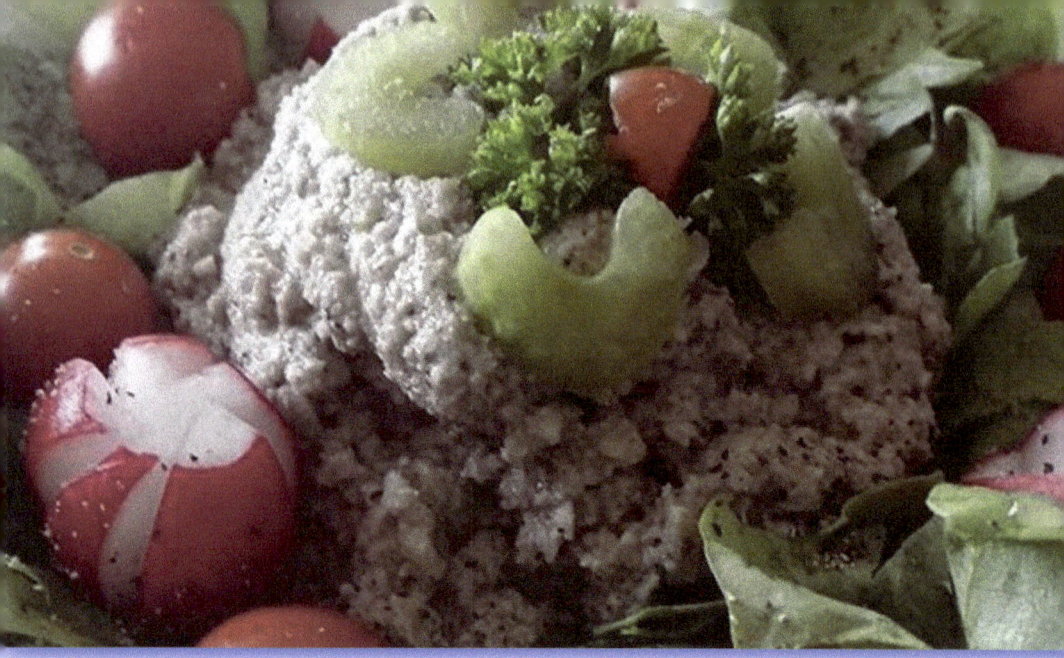

"Tuna" Salad

Preparation: 15 Min.
Soaking: 8-12 Hrs.
Makes 6-8 Servings

Ingredients

"Tuna"

- 1 c. sunflower seeds soaked overnight
- ¼ c. onion, minced
- Himalayan crystal salt to taste
- 1 lemon, juiced
- 2 stocks of celery
- 1 tbsp. kelp
- 1 zucchini

Salad

- 2 c. lettuce
- ½ c. radishes
- ¼ c. celery
- 1 avocado, sliced
- 2 tomatoes, sliced

Directions

Soak sunflower seeds overnight. Drain water and rinse. Place the seeds in food processor.

Cut celery into half inch pieces. Add celery, onion, salt, lemon juice, zucchini and kelp to food processor and blend. It should be roughly mixed.

Wash and tear lettuce into bite-sized pieces and palace on a plate. Scoop about 1/2 cup of the tuna onto the center of the plate. Place radishes and tomatoes around. May use sliced avocado if you wish. Place a few slices of celery on the top of the tuna.

Variations

Instead of using sunflower seeds try walnuts or mix of both then mix as directed. If no zucchini is available may use ¾ c. nut mayo in place.

Brussels Sprout Hazelnut Salad

Preparation: 20 Min. Makes 4-6 Servings

Ingredients

- 1 c. Brussels sprouts
- ½ c. hazelnuts
- 1 tbsp. olive oil
- 1 tsp. coconut nectar
- 1 ½ tsp. thyme
- ½ tsp. Himalayan crystal salt
- ¼ tsp. black pepper
- 2 tbsp. basil
- 2 tsp. turmeric

Fun Fact

Peak season for Brussels sprouts is late September to February.

Directions

Cut hazelnuts in half and soak overnight. Drain water off hazelnuts.

Wash and tear leaves off Brussels sprouts and place in a bowl.

To Brussels sprouts add olive oil, lemon juice, coconut nectar, thyme, salt, pepper, basil, and turmeric toss until everything is well coated and let marinate for at least an hour. Mix hazelnuts with Brussels sprout leaves.

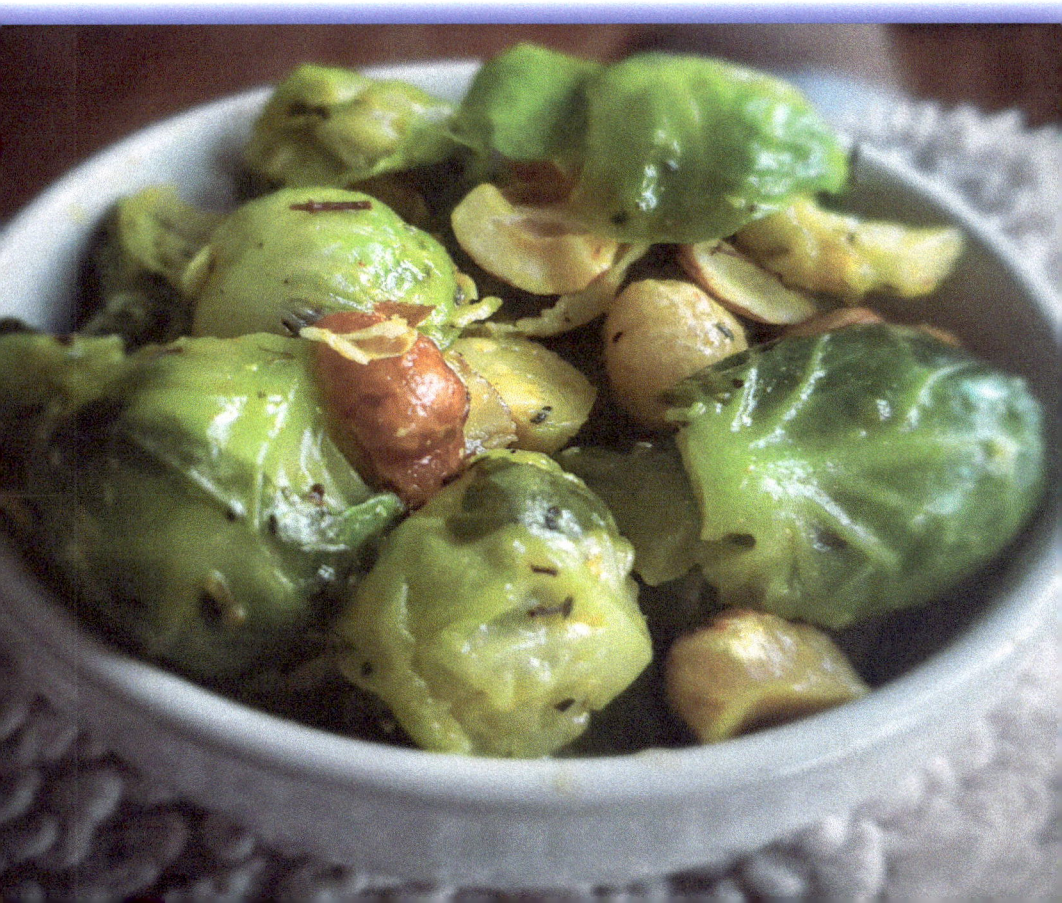

Greek Salad

Preparation: 25 Min.
Makes 2-4 Servings

Ingredients

Salad

- 1 head crisp lettuce, torn into bite sized pieces
- 1 red bell pepper, sliced
- 4 tomatoes cut into wedges
- 1 red onion, sliced into rings
- sundried olives (optional)
- ½ c. vegan basil feta cheese (page 149, optional)

Greek Dressing

- ½ c raw tahini
- 1 lemon, juiced
- ½ tsp. ground cumin
- ½ tsp. paprika
- 1 clove garlic
- 4 tbsp. cold pressed olive oil
- ½ c. pure water
- pinch Himalayan crystal salt

Directions

Make vegan basil feta cheese and set aside.

Slice bell pepper, red onion, and chop tomatoes place in a large bowl. Tear lettuce into bite-sized pieces and toss with the bell peppers.

In a blender, place tahini, olive oil, lemon juice, cumin, paprika, garlic, salt, and water blend until creamy. Pour the dressing over the salad.

Crumble feta and sliced olives over the top.

> **Fun Fact**
>
> The ancient Greeks and Romans thought that eating lettuce helped you to have a good night's sleep.

Strawberry Kiwi Salad

Preparation: 5 Min.
Makes 2 Servings

Ingredients

- 1 banana
- ¾ c. strawberries
- 2 kiwi
- ¼ c. dried coconut (optional)

Directions

Peel and slice kiwi and banana placing in a bowl. Wash and slice strawberries and add to kiwi and banana. Sprinkle with coconut if desired.

> **Fun Fact**
>
> Kiwi fruit contains two times more vitamin C than oranges. They are also a rich source of vitamin E and K.

Creamy Lemon Poppy Seed Dressing

Preparation: 5 Min. *Makes 4-6 Servings*

Ingredients

- 1 c. cashews
- 2 lemons, juiced
- 2 tsp. organic lemon zest
- ½ tsp. mustard seed, ground
- 1 tsp. stevia leaves
- 1 tsp. Himalayan crystal salt
- 2 tbsp. poppy seeds
- ½ c. water

Directions

Place cashews into a blender add lemon juice, lemon zest, make sure the lemon zest is organic, add ground mustard seed, stevia leaves, salt, and mix until smooth. Add water as needed until the desired constancy is achieved.

Remove dressing from blender and place in a bowl. Stir in poppy seeds and serve.

Strawberry Dressing

Preparation: 20 Min. *Makes 2-4 Servings*

Ingredients

- ¾ c. fresh strawberries
- 2 tbsp. lime juice
- 1 tsp. raw apple cider vinegar
- 4 tsp. coconut nectar
- 1 tsp. poppy seeds
- Himalayan crystal salt
- white pepper to taste

Directions

Combine strawberries with lime juice, raw apple cider vinegar, and the coconut nectar in a blender.

Add salt, pepper and poppy seeds and blend until well combined.

Variation

For Cherry Dressing omit strawberry juice and replace with cherry juice.

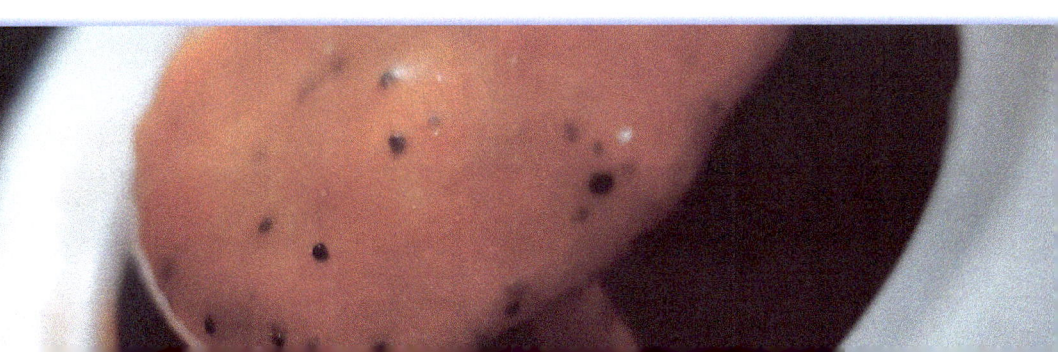

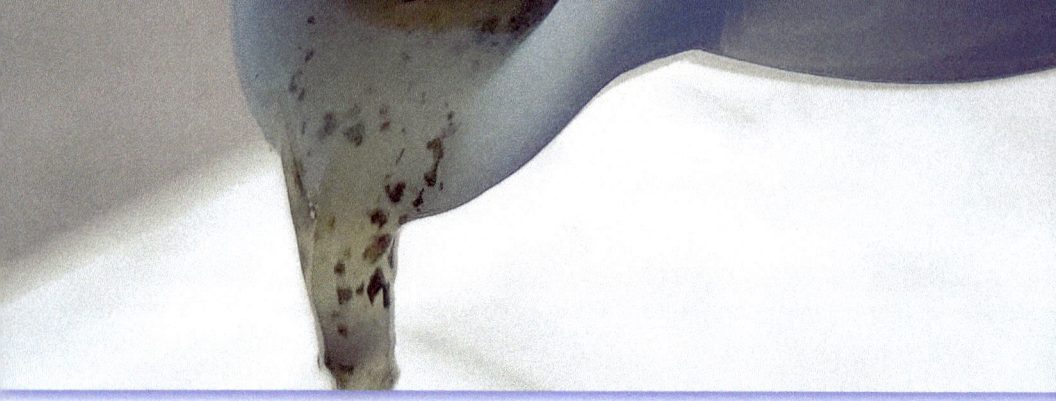

Italian Dressing

Preparation: 15 Min. Makes 2-4 Servings

Ingredients

- 3 tbsp. cold pressed olive oil
- 1 tsp. raw apple cider vinegar
- 1 tbsp. fresh parsley
- 4 tbsp. fresh lemon juice
- 1 cloves garlic
- 1 tbsp. fresh basil
- ¼ tsp. crushed red pepper
- ½ tbsp. fresh oregano

Directions

Finely chop parsley, basil, garlic, and oregano then place in a bowl. To the spices combine oil, vinegar, lemon juice, and crushed red pepper whisk until well mixed.

You can also place ingredients in a jar with a lid and shake

Variation

For a winter dressing use ½ tsp. each of dried parsley, basil, oregano and garlic powder or 1 tablespoon of Italian seasoning.

Tangy Tomato Dressing

Preparation: 15 Min. Makes 2-4 Servings

Ingredients

- 2 c. tomatoes
- 1 tbsp. raw apple cider vinegar
- Himalayan crystal salt to taste
- white pepper to taste
- 1 c. dried tomato
- ¼ tsp. onion powder
- Pinch cayenne pepper
- ¼ tsp. paprika
- ¼ hot pepper

Directions

Cut tomatoes and place in a blender, add raw apple cider vinegar, salt, pepper, and dried tomatoes.

Cut and seed the hot pepper and add it to the blender. Combine along with paprika, onion power, and cayenne pepper blend until smooth.

Simple Salsa

Preparation: 15 Min.   Makes 2-4 Servings

Ingredients

- 2 c. tomato chopped
- ½ onion, chopped
- 3 cloves garlic
- ¼ c. cilantro
- Himalayan crystal salt

Directions

Place tomato, onion, garlic, cilantro, and salt in a food processor. Pulse until very coarsely chopped.

Party Dip

Preparation: 15 Min.   Soaking: 8-12 Hrs.   Makes 2-4 Servings

Ingredients

- sunflower beans (page 56)
- spicy cheese (page 146)
- guacamole (page 59)
- sour cream (page 144)
- 3-4 green onions, finely chopped.
- 1 bell pepper (yellow, red, orange or a combination of), chopped
- 1 large tomato, chopped

Note

For winter omit bell pepper and tomato or use dried.

Directions

Make sunflower beans, spicy cheese, guacamole and sour cream.

Spread sunflower beans in pan. Dehydrate for a few hours, if desired.

Take out beans out and layer spicy cheese, guacamole, green onions, bell peppers, and tomato. Top with sour cream. Serve with favorite cracker or eat as a casserole.

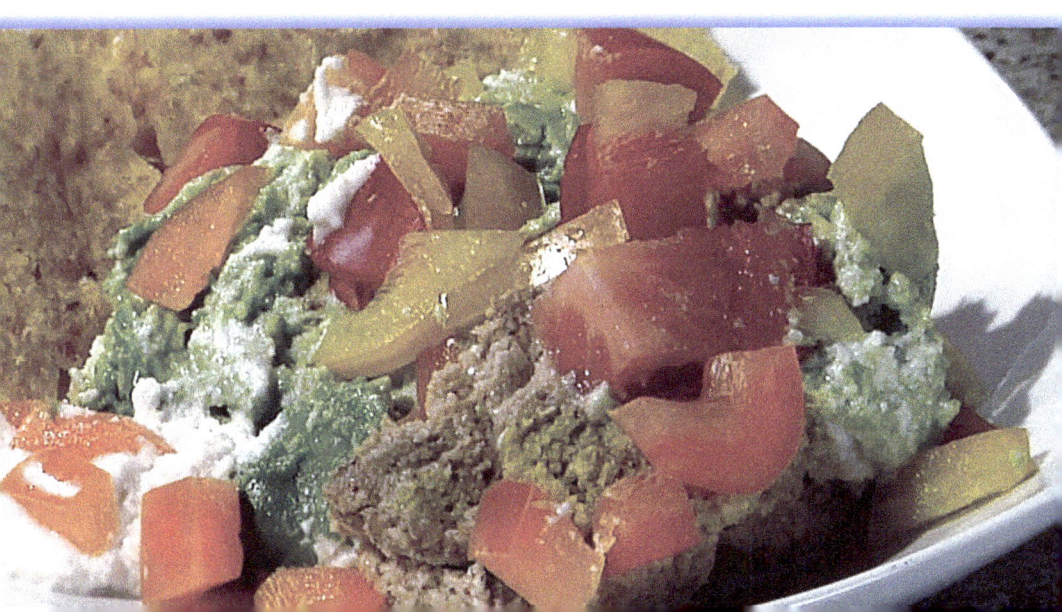

Onion Dip

Preparation: 15 Min. *Makes 2-4 Servings*

Ingredients

- 2 c. almonds, soaked and pealed
- 1 garlic clove
- ¼ c. onion
- 2 tbsp. dill
- 1 lemon, juiced
- 1 c. pure water
- 1 tsp. Himalayan crystal salt to taste
- ¼ c. green onion
- 1 tbsp. parsley
- 1 tbsp. raw apple cider vinegar
- 1 tbsp. cold pressed olive oil
- 1 tsp. white pepper

Directions

Soak almonds overnight, while wet, peel brown skins off.

In a blender, combine almond, garlic, onion, garlic, dill, lemon juice, salt, green onion, parsley, vinegar, olive oil, and pepper blend until well combined using only enough water to achieve thickness desired.

> **Fun Fact**
>
> During the Middle Ages, onions were used as gifts and currency.

Beet Hummus

Preparation: 15 Min. *Makes 2-4 Servings*

Ingredients

- 2 c. cashews
- 2 cloves garlic cloves
- 1 tbsp. raw tahini
- 1 lemon, juiced
- 1 tsp. Himalayan crystal salt
- ½ c. beets
- 2 tbsp. cold pressed olive oil (optional)

Variation

Replace cashews for sprouted garbanzo beans.

Directions

Soak cashews for about 15 minutes. Soaking soften the nuts and makes them easier to cream. However, this recipe will work if you skip this step. Drain water off cashews and place them in food processor.

Chop beet and place in a food processor with cashews and mix until smooth. Add, garlic, tahini, salt, lemon and olive oil continue blending until well mixed.

Serve with raw crackers or veggies.

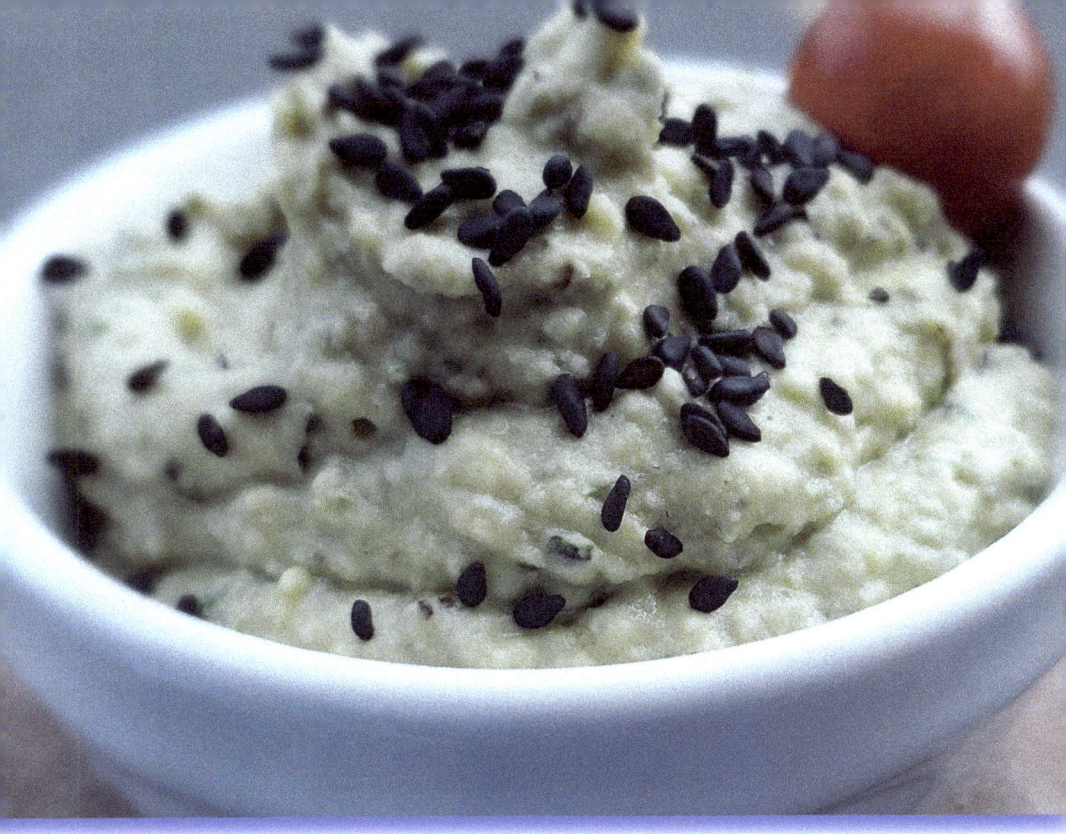

Kale Hummus

Preparation: 15 Min. Sprouting: 3-5 Days Makes 6-8 Servings

Ingredients

- handful kale
- 2 c. garbanzo beans, sprouted
- 1 cloves garlic clove
- 2 tbsp. raw tahini
- 1 tsp. organic lemon zest
- 1 lemon, juiced
- 1 tsp. Himalayan crystal salt
- 2 tbsp. cold pressed olive oil
- 1 tsp. black sesame seeds (optional)

Variation

Replace garbanzo beans with soaked and peeled almonds.

Directions

Sprout garbanzo beans, they should be soft and easily smashed with a fork, about 2-6 days.

Wash kale and remove steams. Use cold pressed olive oil and massage or rub it into kale. Place the kale in a food processor add garbanzo beans, garlic, tahini, salt, lemon, and lemon zest mix until smooth and well mixed.

Sprinkle with black sesame seeds. Serve with raw crackers or veggies.

Carrot Hummus

Preparation: *Soaking:*   *Makes 6-8*
15 Min.   *8-12 Hrs.*   *Servings*

Ingredients

- 3 carrots
- 2 c. almonds, soaked and peeled
- 1 clove garlic
- 5 tbsp. raw tahini
- 1 tsp. thyme
- 1 tsp. sesame seed
- 1 ½ tsp. Himalayan crystal salt
- 1 lemon, juiced
- 2 tbsp. cold pressed olive oil

Directions

Soak almonds overnight. Peel off brown skin while still wet.

Chop carrots and place in a food processor and pulse until smooth. Add almonds, garlic, clove, tahini, thyme, sesame seed, salt, lemon and olive oil mix until smooth and well mixed.

Serve with raw crackers or veggies.

Variation

Replace almonds with sprouted garbanzo beans.

Sunflower Beans

Preparation: *Soaking:*   *Makes 4-6*
15 Min.   *8-12 Hrs.*   *Servings*

Ingredients

- 2½ c. sunflower seeds, soaked overnight
- ¼ c. cold pressed olive oil
- 3 ½ tsp. onion powder
- 1 tbsp. chili powder
- 2 tsp. cumin seed powder
- 1 tsp. Himalayan crystal salt
- 1 tbsp. raw apple cider vinegar
- ¼ c. onion, chopped
- 1 bell pepper (your choice color and combination
- 1 hot pepper if desired.
- pure water if needed

Directions

Soak sunflower seeds overnight. Drain off water and place seeds into food processor. Cut bell peppers, onion, and hot pepper place in food processor with sunflower seeds. Add olive oil, spice, and vinegar combined until smooth adding only enough water to ensure consistency.

For people who are not used to raw foods, I recommend warming the beans in a dehydrator for an hour or so at 100°F.

Taco Meat

Preparation: 30 Min. *Makes 4-6 Servings*

Ingredients

- 2 c. butternut squash
- 1-2 tsp. chili powder
- 2-3 tsp. Himalayan crystal salt
- ½ tsp. Mexican seasoning
- 2 hot peppers
- ¼ c. onion

Directions

Peel, seed, and shred squash. Place squash, chili powder, salt, Mexican seasoning, onion, and hot peppers in a food processor, combine until it is chunky and looks a little like ground meat.

Ground Meatless

Preparation: 10 Min. *Soaking: 6-8 Hrs.* *Makes 4-6 Servings*

Ingredients

- 2 c. walnuts, soaked
- 1 tsp. poultry seasoning
- 1 tsp. Italian seasoning
- 1 clove garlic
- 4 tbsp. onion
- ½ tsp. Himalayan crystal salt
- ½ c. carrots, chopped (optional)

Directions

Soak walnuts overnight. Drain water off and place walnuts in a food processor.

To food processor add carrot, garlic, poultry seasoning, Italian seasoning, salt and onion. Mix until it is chunky and looks a little like ground meat.

Basic Pâté

Preparation: 10 Min. *Soaking: 8-12 Hrs.* *Makes 6-8 Servings*

Ingredients

- 2 c. favorite nut or seeds
- ½ onion, chopped
- 2 tsp. parsley
- 2 cloves garlic, minced
- ¼ c. lemon, juiced
- ¼ c. cold pressed olive oil
- Himalayan crystal salt
- white pepper to taste

Directions

Soak preferred nut or seed overnight. Drain off water and place nut/seed in food processor. Add onion, garlic, lemon juice, olive oil, parsley, salt, and pepper combine until pâté texture is achieved.

Use for dipping vegetables or on a salad or as a filling. I use it to stuff bell peppers.

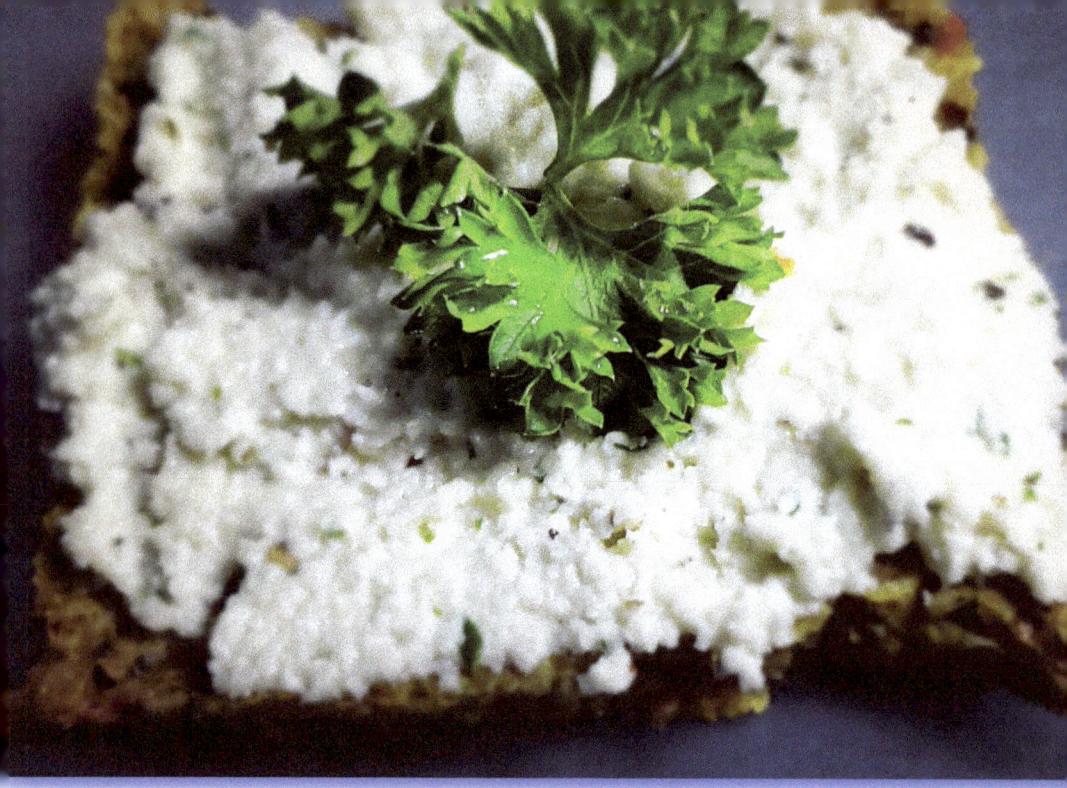

Herbed Almond Spread

Preparation: 15 Min.   Soaking: 8-12 Hrs.   Makes 2-4 Servings

Ingredients

- 1 c. walnuts, soaked & dried
- 1 lemon, juiced
- ½ c. almonds, soaked overnight
- 1-2 tbsp. garlic powder
- ¼ tsp. Himalayan crystal salt
- ¼ c. cold pressed olive oil
- 1 tsp. mustard powder
- ¼ c parsley, minced
- ¼ c. pure water

Directions

Soak walnuts and almonds overnight. Drain off water and place nuts, garlic, and salt in a food processor and mix until roughly mixed.

Add lemon juice, garlic, salt, oil, mustard powder, and parsley. Blend until it resembles a thick paste adding only enough water as needed to achieve a smooth texture.

Use the almond spread on crackers or as a veggie dip.

Fun Fact

The almond is botanically a stone fruit related to cherry, plum, peach and apricot.

Guacamole

Preparation: 5 Min. *Makes 4-6 Servings*

Ingredients

- ¼ c. nut mayo (page 143)
- 1-2 large avocadoes
- Himalayan crystal salt to taste

Directions

Make mayo. Cut avocadoes in half, remove seed and peel. Place avocado flesh in a bowl and combine with salt and mayo with a fork until blended.

Salsa

Preparation: 15 Min. *Makes 4-6 Servings*

Ingredients

- 1 yellow bell pepper
- 1 red bell pepper, chopped
- 1 orange bell pepper
- 2 hot peppers, chopped
- 1 c. onion, chopped
- 4-5 fresh tomatoes
- 1 cloves garlic, minced
- 1 lime, juiced

Directions

Wash and chop onion, tomatoes, hot pepper, garlic, yellow, orange and red bell peppers. In a bowl combine all the chopped vegetables along with lime juice.

This can be done in a food processor and pulse but be careful because it can easily turn into soup.

Carrot Mushroom Stir-fry

Preparation: 20 Min. *Marinating: 2-12 Hrs.* *Makes 4-6 Servings*

Ingredients

- 7 medium carrots
- 2-4 tbsp. cold pressed olive oil
- 2 tsp. Himalayan crystal salt
- 1 tsp. turmeric
- 1 c. mushrooms
- 5 green onions
- ½ lemon or lime, juiced
- ¼ tsp. black pepper, ground

Directions

Thinly slice carrots, green onion and mushrooms, place in a bowl. In a jar with a lid place olive oil, salt, 2 tbsp. lemon juice, and turmeric with lid on shake jar until well mixed.

Pour dressing over vegetables and mix until everything is well coated. Marinate one hour. Just before serving, add reaming lemon juice and pepper. Toss and serve. May be warmed to 100°F

Sauerkraut

Preparation: 15 Min. Fermenting: 1-2 Weeks. Makes 2-4 Servings

Ingredients

- 1 head organic cabbage,
- 1 small onion, thinly sliced
- 1 tbsp. dill
- 3 tbsp. Himalayan crystal salt

Directions

Shred cabbage using a mandolin or food processor with the grater on.

Place shredded cabbage in a large pan. Mix cabbage onion, dill, and salt with your hands. Pack gently with hands or potato masher. Repeat until pan is nearly full, about 2 inches from the top.

Cover with cloth, and place a plate with clean rocks or something heavy on top. During the curing process, sauerkraut needs daily attention. It will form liquid brine.

Remove scum as it forms and wash or replace cloth often to keep it free from scum and mold. At room temperature, fermentation will be completed in 10 to 12 days.

Pack into jars adding enough liquid to fill jars. If there is not enough liquid to fill the jar make a weak brine by dissolving 2 tablespoons of salt to a quart of water.

Traditionally green cabbage is used to make sauerkraut, but red cabbage can be used.

Note

Always use **organic cabbage** when making sauerkraut. Cabbage is a crop that is highly treated with sprays. Fermenting will intensify the chemicals that were used to spray the cabbage.

Fun Fact

Raw cabbage is very rich in vitamin C. Sauerkraut is also an excellent source of Vitamin K. In the old times, Vitamin C was hard to come by during the winter.

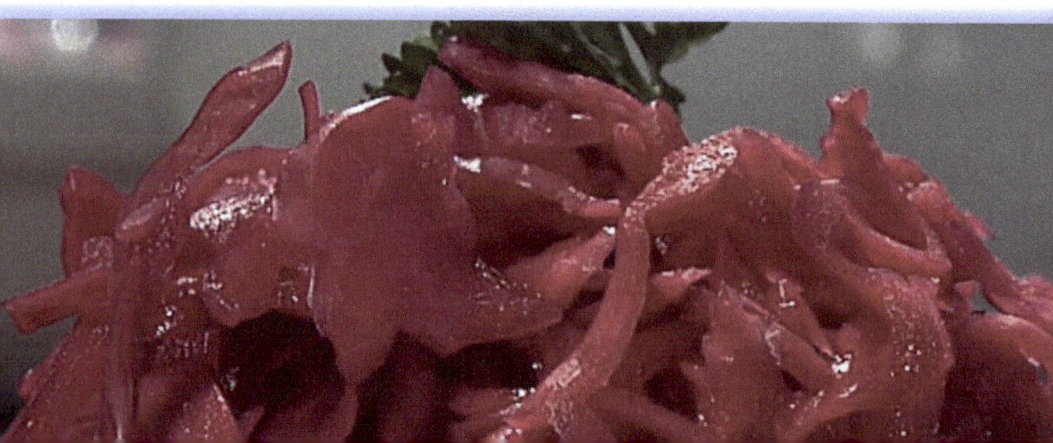

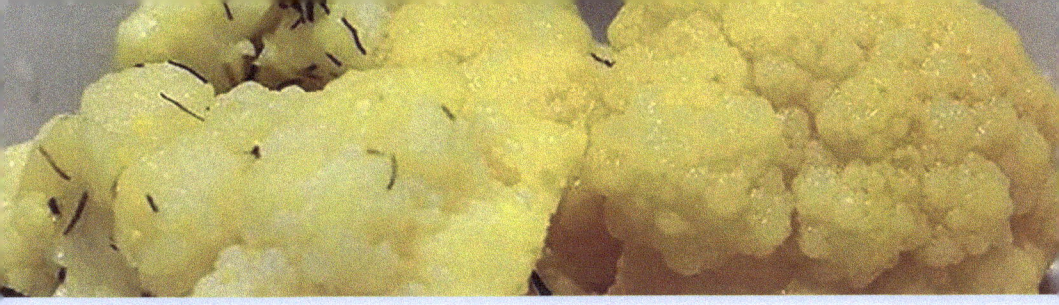

Pickled Cauliflower

Preparation: 30 Min.

Fermenting: 3-10 Days

Makes 1-2 Quarts

Ingredients

- 1 ½ c. filtered water
- 1 ½ tsp. Himalayan crystal salt
- 1 small cauliflower head, any color
- ¾ tsp. turmeric
- 4-8 springs of fresh dill
- 3 cloves garlic
- 1 tsp. celery seed
- 1 tsp. coriander seed
- 1 tsp. mustard seed
- ½ tsp. black peppercorn

Note

1. It takes about 3-10 days before cauliflower is ready, depending on the temperature and how sour you like them. Taste them from time to time to test taste and texture. When they taste good to you, they are done.

2. Store cauliflower it in the refrigerator with tight lid. Because there is no vinegar to preserve the cauliflower, they will keep about 2 weeks.

Directions

Prepare salt brine by combining filtered water and salt. When salt dissolves the brine is ready.

In a jar place turmeric, dill, garlic, celery seed, coriander seed, mustard seed and peppercorn. Wash cauliflower then separate into small florets. Tightly pack cauliflower florets into the jar.

Pour salt brine into jar. It should completely cover the cauliflower. Set the lid loosely on top of the jar; don't seal it. Cover with the clean dish towel and put jar in the pantry or cupboard, or in a warm (65°F to 75°F), dark place where it won't be disturbed.

After about 2 days, start to visually inspect the water in the jar to see if it has bubbles rising to the top. The water will become cloudy and there may be a scum forming on the top of the water. This is normal and not a problem; simply scoop away the scum with a clean spoon that has been rinsed with filtered (non-chlorinated) water.

Cauliflower may begin to smell a little sour, which is fine, but if the smell is rotten, something might have gone wrong and it may need to be thrown out.

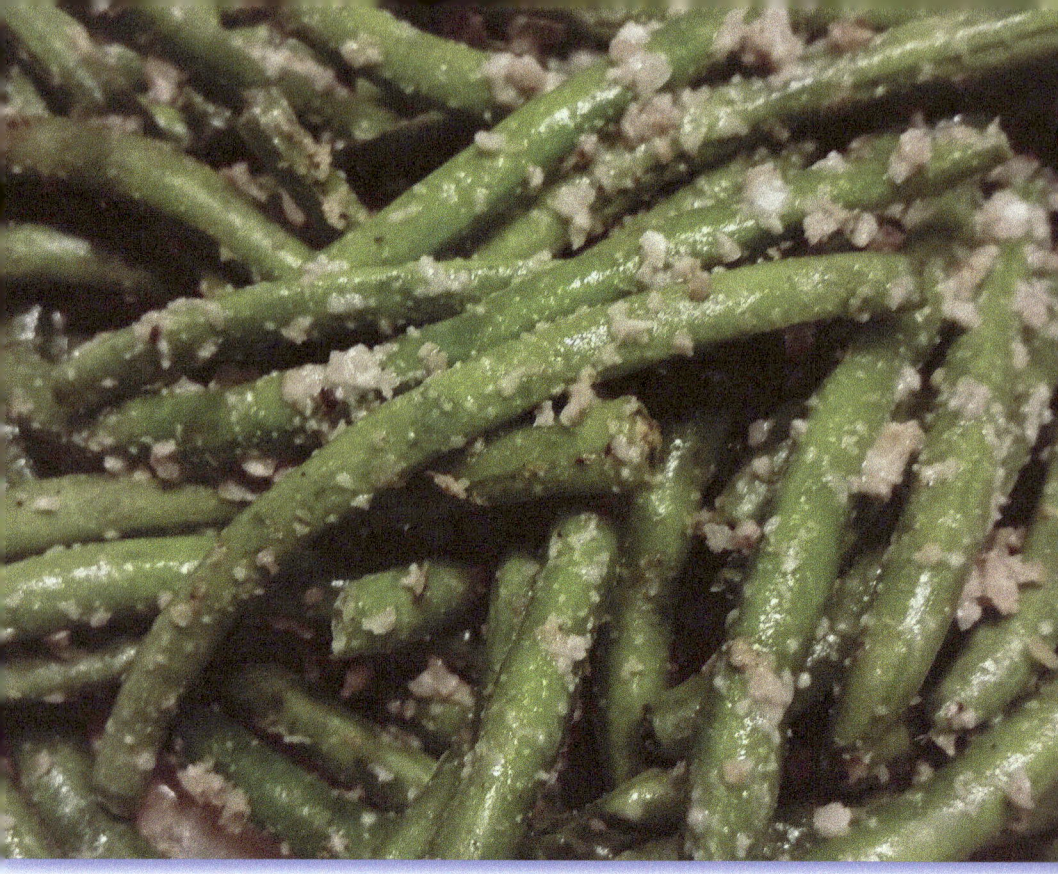

Georgian Green Beans

Preparation: 15 Min.
Soaking: 1-8 Hrs
Drying: 1-2 Hrs
Makes 4-6 Servings

Ingredients

- 3 c. fresh green beans
- ¼ c. walnuts, soaked overnight
- 1 clove garlic
- pinch of cayenne pepper
- 1 tbsp. raw apple cider vinegar
- 3 tbsp. water
- ½ tsp. Himalayan crystal salt
- 2 tbsp. sweet red or white onion, finely chopped

Directions

Soak walnuts overnight. Drain water off and place into a blender. Add garlic, cayenne pepper, vinegar, salt, onion, and water to the walnuts and blend until smooth.

Cut green beans into 1 inch pieces. Pour blended mixture over green beans and stir. Make sure to cover all of the green beans. Chill for at least an hour, the longer the flavors mingle, the better it will taste.

If you desire a more cooked feeling, dehydrate 2 hours before serving.

Snappy Vegetables

Preparation: 20 Min. *Makes 4-6 Servings*

Ingredients

- 2 c. sugar snap peas
- 1 red bell pepper
- 1 zucchini squash
- 1 cloves garlic, minced
- 1 lemon, juiced
- 1 tbsp. Italian seasoning
- 1 head lettuce
- ½ c. macadamia nuts or cashews, grated

Directions

Wash and remove string from snap peas. Slice bell pepper and zucchini then place in a bowl with snap peas.

In a separate bowl or jar with a lid, combine lemon oil, Italian seasoning, and minced garlic until well mixed. Pour dressing over vegetables and toss together.

Line a serving plate with lettuce, place vegetables over greens. Use the grated macadamia nuts as "cheese" and sprinkle over top.

Fun Fact

Sugar snap peas are a cross between English and snow peas. They were developed in the 17th century.

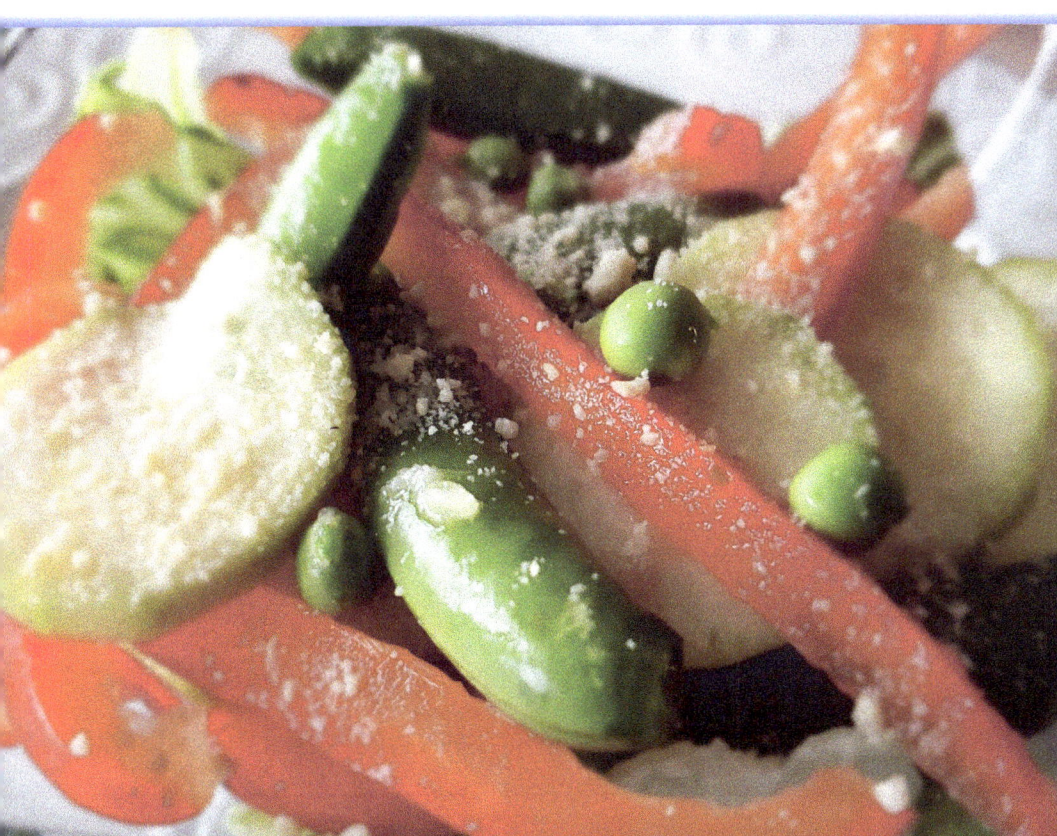

Spicy Jicama Fries

Preparation: 25 Min.   Sprouting: 3-5 days   Makes 6-8 Servings

Ingredients

- 1 large jicama
- ¾ tbsp. onion powder
- 1 tbsp. cold pressed olive oil
- 1 ½ tsp. chili seasoning
- ½ tsp. garlic powder
- pinch cayenne
- ½ lemon, juiced

Directions

Peel and slice the jicama into sticks (like a French fries).

Place in a container with a tight-fitting lid. Add onion powder, garlic powder, cayenne, chili seasoning, lemon juice and olive oil. Put lid on and shake until jicama is well coated.

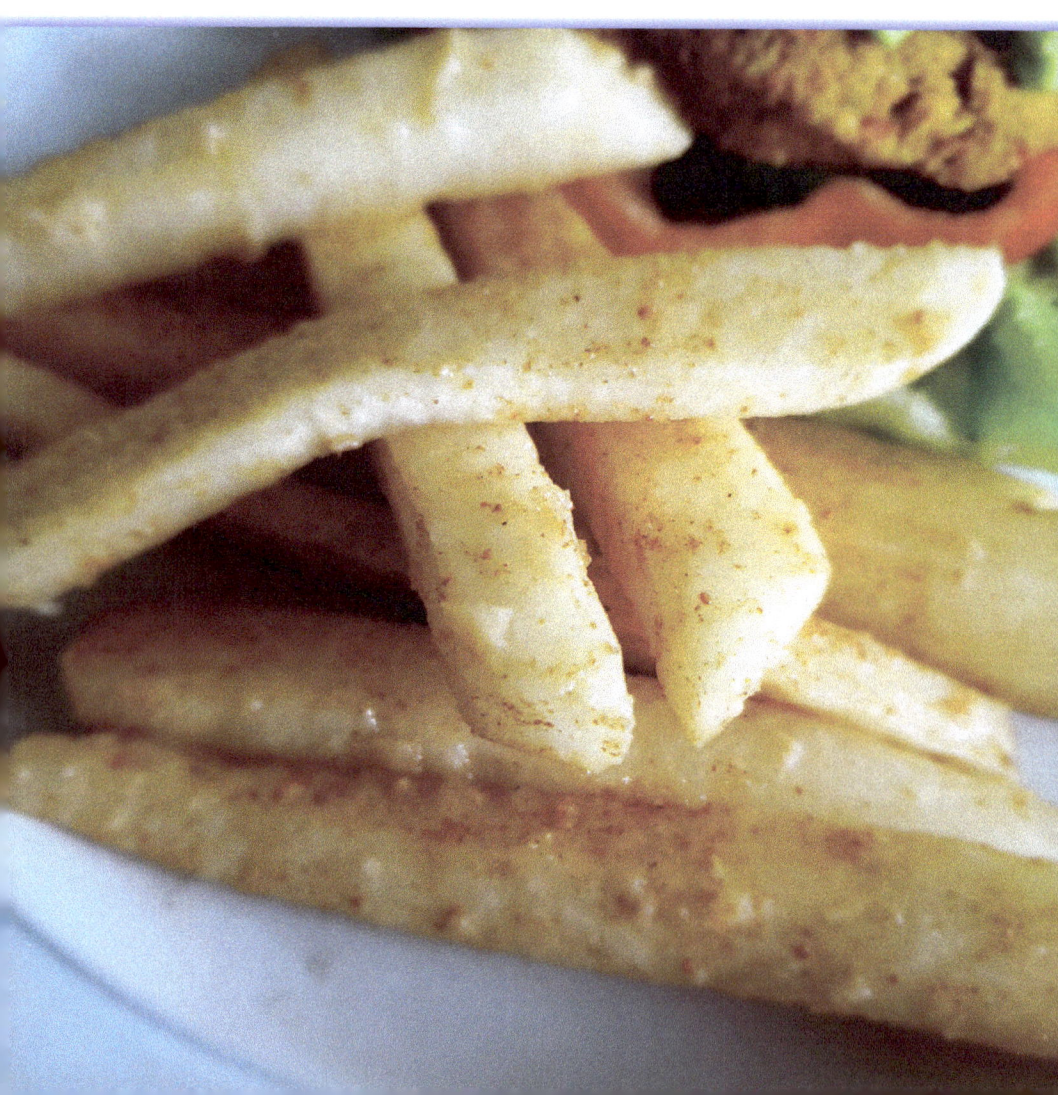

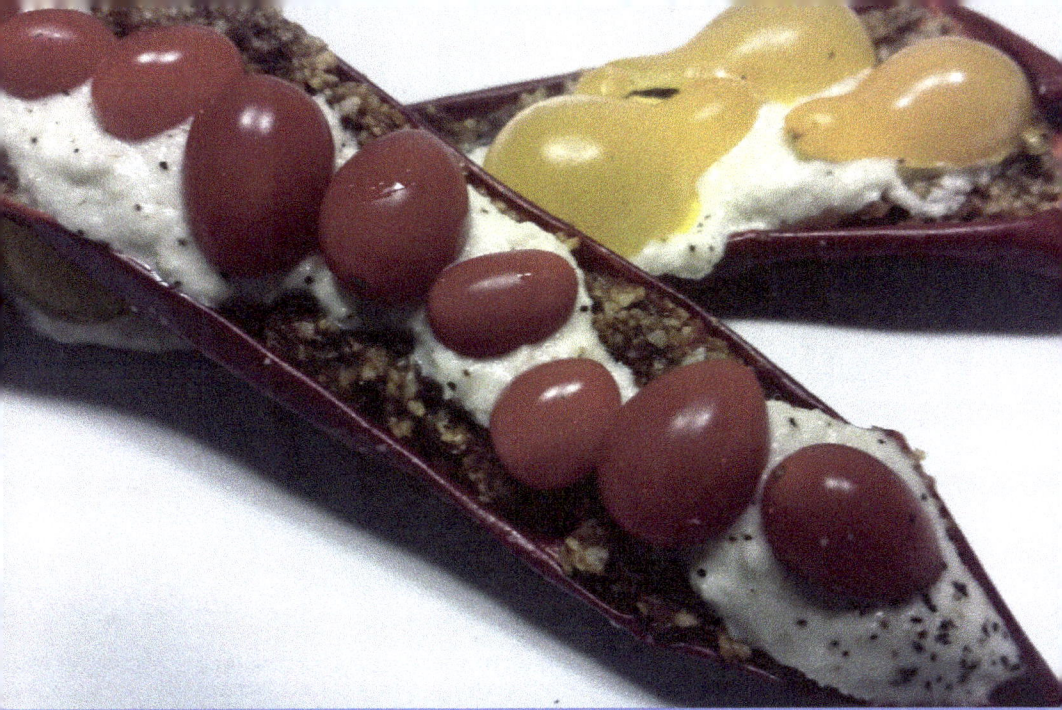

Stuffed Anaheim Peppers

Preparation: 20 Min. *Drying:* 4-8 Hrs. *Makes 4-6 Servings*

Ingredients

- 6 Anaheim peppers
- sunflower beans (page 56)
- sour cream (page 144)
- tomatoes, chopped
- guacamole (page 59, optional)

Note

For winter use dried pepper and tomatoes.

Directions

Make sunflower beans. Cut Anaheim peppers lengthwise in half and remove the seeds and wash.

Stuff peppers with beans. Dehydrate for about 3 hours at 100°F or until warm and desired Anaheim texture is achieved.

Serve with a dab of sour cream and guacamole; top with a few chopped tomatoes, cherry tomatoes or salsa. Add salt and pepper to taste before serving.

Fun Fact

Anaheim peppers are normally very mild only 500 to 2,500 on the Scoville heat scale making it about eight times milder than the average jalapeno.

Nadhirrah's Jalapeño Poppers

| Preparation: | Soaking: | Drying: | Makes 6-8 |
| 15 Min. | 8-12 Hrs. | 12-24 Hrs. | Servings |

Ingredients

- 1-pound jalapenos
- 2-3 c. orange, juiced
- ½ c. sour cream (page 144)

Stuffing

- 1 c. pumpkins seed soaked
- 1 tsp. cold pressed olive oil
- 2 lemons, juiced
- ½ tsp. Himalayan crystal salt
- 1 tsp. dried dill or a little more fresh
- 2 green onions, chopped
- ½ red bell pepper
- ½ c. tomato, chopped

Note

It is a good idea to wear gloves when dealing with jalapeños and do not touch your face after touching the jalapeño.

Directions

Soak pumpkins seeds overnight. Slice jalapenos in the middle and remove the seeds and place in a bowl.

Squeeze 3 cups of oranges juice or enough to cover jalapenos in the bowl. Soak jalapenos overnight in orange juice.

Drain water off of pumpkin seeds and place in a food processor add olive oil, lemon juice, salt, dill, green onions, bell pepper, and tomato combine until well mixed. This can be made ahead of time and sit while the peppers are marinating.

On a mesh sheet dehydrator tray arranged the peppers. Fill each pepper with stuffing. Dehydrate at 110°F until they are the consistency you like. Usually about 12 to 24 hours. Drizzle with sour cream.

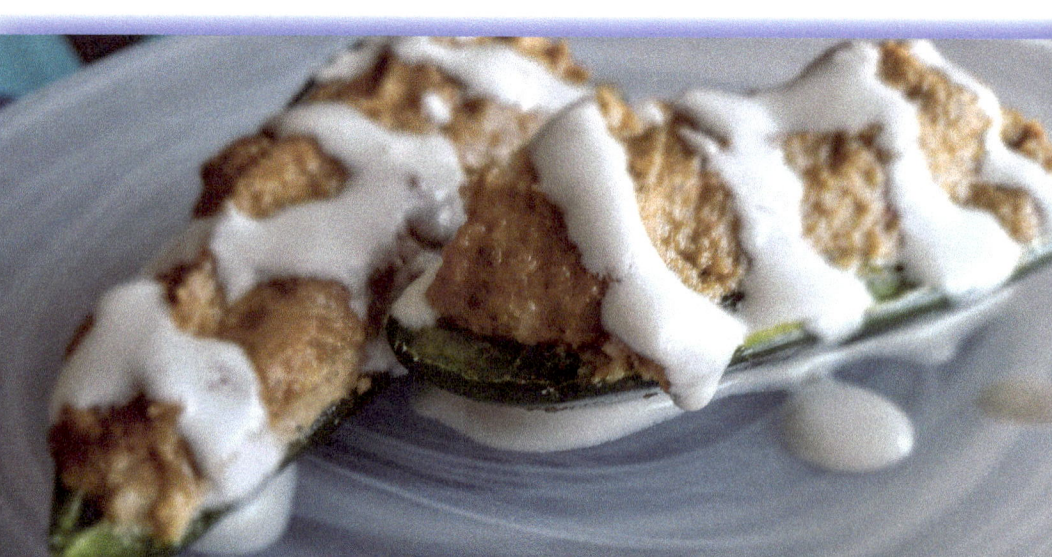

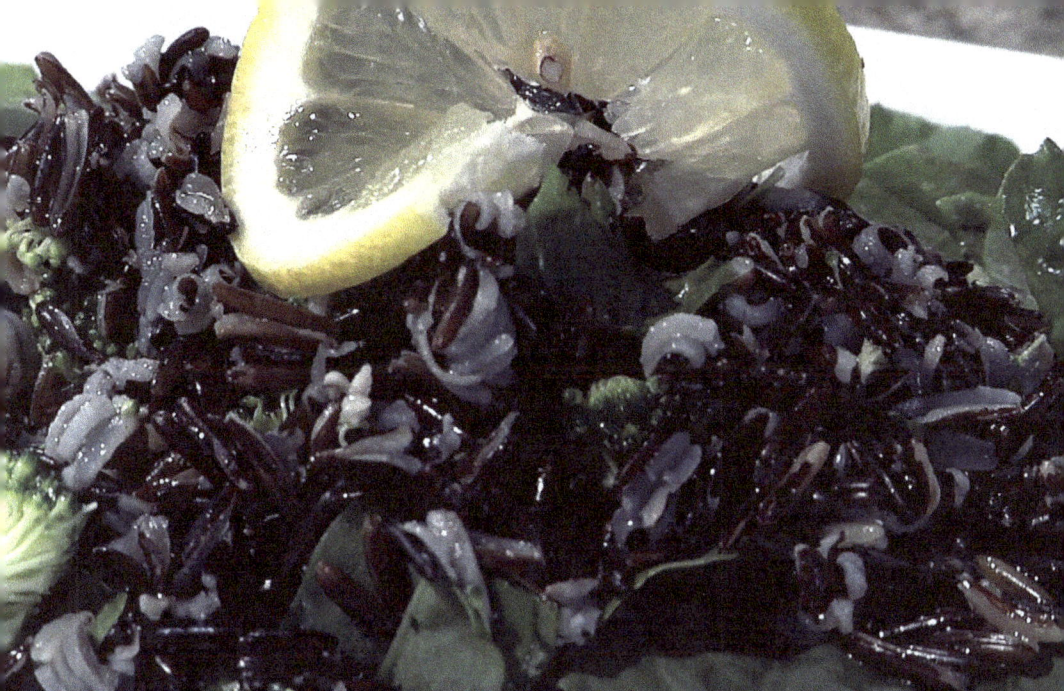

Lemon Rice

Ingredients

- 2 c. wild rice, sprouted
- ½ c. onion, finely chopped
- 2 tsp. cold pressed olive oil
- 1 ½ lemons, juiced
- ¼ tsp. Himalayan crystal salt
- 2 c. fresh spinach, chopped
- 1 ½ c. broccoli, chopped

Preparation: 15 Min.

Soaking: 2-3 Days

Makes 2-4 Servings

Directions

Sprout rice (page 13). In a bowl combine onion, olive oil, lemon juice, salt, spinach, broccoli, and rice.

Set aside to allow flavors to mingle. May warm if desired.

Note

Lemon spinach is the best for this recipe.

Fun Facts

Wild Rice is not a grain but a grass seed from a different botanical family.

Wild rice has about twice the protein of other rice, provides about 50% of the recommended daily allowance of folascin, 40% niacin, and 20% vitamin B6.

Wild Jambalaya

Preparation: 45 Min.   Sprouting: 1-3 Days   Makes 6-8 Servings

Ingredients

- 2 c. wild rice, sprouted

Sauce

- 1-2 cloves garlic
- 2 ½ c. tomatoes
- 1 tsp. oregano, dried
- 1 tbsp. fresh parsley or 1 tsp. dried
- 1 tsp. thyme
- ¼ - ½ small hot pepper
- dash paprika
- ½ tsp. pepper
- ½ tsp. Himalayan crystal salt
- ¼ c. sun-dried tomatoes

Vegetables

- 1 medium red bell pepper,
- 1 medium onion, finely
- 2 medium tomatoes, finely
- 1 c. zucchini
- ½ c. celery
- 1 c. broccoli florets

Directions

Sprout wild rice (page 13) and set aside.

In a blender, mix garlic, tomatoes, oregano, parsley, thyme, hot pepper, paprika, pepper salt and sun-dried tomatoes until well mixed.

Chop bell pepper, onion, tomatoes, zucchini, celery and broccoli mix in a bowl.

Pour blender sauce over vegetables and mix. Stir in rice and serve right away or let sit for a couple of hours.

Fun Fact

There are two main types of jambalaya. The Creole method contains tomatoes while the Southwestern and South Central Louisiana jambalaya is tomato free.

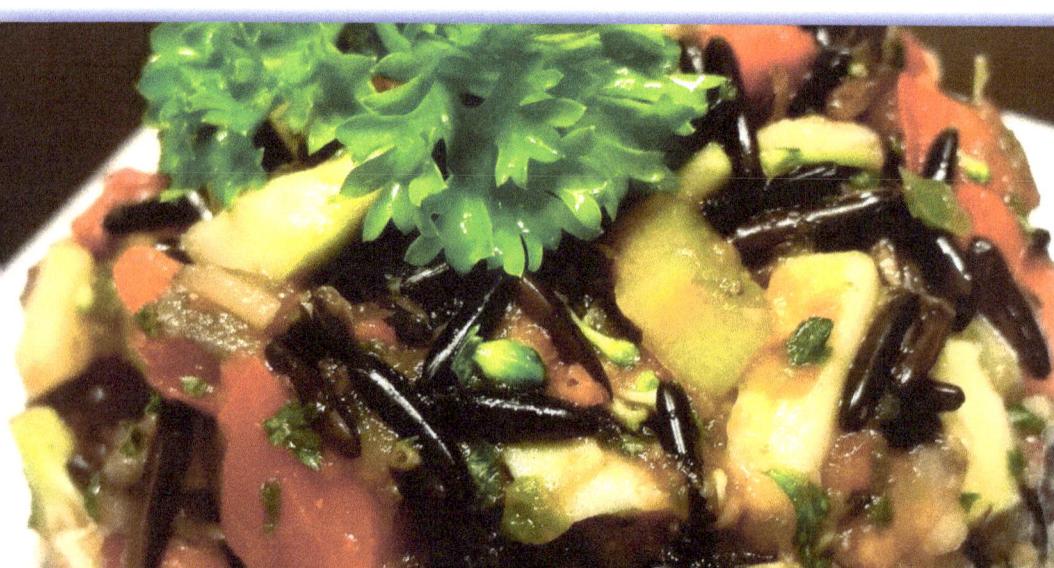

Dirty Rice

Preparation: 20 Min.
Sprouting: 1-3 days
Makes 6-8 Servings

Ingredients

- 1 tsp. cold pressed olive oil
- 1 small onion, chopped
- 1 stalk celery, thinly sliced
- ½ c. red bell pepper
- 1 clove garlic, minced
- 3 c. wild rice, sprouted
- 1 ½ c. mixed sprouts
- ½ c. peas
- 1 tbsp. thyme
- 1 tsp. cumin, ground
- ½ tsp. cayenne pepper
- 1 c. spinach, chopped
- 1 sweet bell Pepper (yellow, orange, or red or combo of the three)
- ½ lime, juiced
- Himalayan crystal salt

Directions

Sprout adzuki beans, green peas, mung beans, fenugreek, use any combination you like. I prefer a mixture of them. Sprout wild rice (page 13).

Chop onion, bell pepper, and spinach. Slice celery and mince garlic then place in a bowl. Add sprouts, rice, peas, olive oil, lime juice, cumin, and cayenne gently mix until everything is well coated. May warm to 100°F if desired.

Fun Fact

The name dirty rice comes from its Cajun origins in Louisiana. Originally, they would throw everything including chicken livers and gizzards into the rice that gave it a "dirty" color. This rice gets its "dirty" color from the herbs and the black rice.

Apple Curry Rice

Preparation: 15 Min.
Sprouting: 1-3 days
Makes 4-6 Servings

Ingredients

- 1 c. black wild rice, sprouted
- 1 tbsp. cold pressed olive oil
- ¼ tsp. curry powder
- 1 small onion, chopped
- 3 medium apples
- 1 garlic clove, minced
- 1 c. peas, fresh or frozen

Directions

Sprout rice (see page 13). Drain water off rice. In a bowl, combine rice, olive oil, curry powder, onion, apples, garlic, and peas. Gently mix together and serve.

Warm Mexi-Rice

Preparation: 20 Min.   Sprouting: 1-3 days   Makes 6-8 Servings

Ingredients

- 2 c. organic wild rice,
- ½ onion
- 1 red bell pepper
- 1 hot pepper
- ½ c. cold pressed olive oil
- 2 tomatoes, chopped
- 2 tbsp. chili powder
- 2 tsp. Himalayan crystal salt
- 1 tsp. turmeric

Directions

Sprout the rice (page 13). Drain water off the rice and place in a bowl.

Chop bell pepper, hot pepper, onion, and tomatoes combine with rice, chili powder, salt and turmeric and gently mix together and serve. May warm to 100°F.

Open Face Tomato Bites

Preparation: 5 Min.   Makes 4-6 Servings

Ingredients

- 4 tbsp. nut mayo (page 143)
- 6 pizza crackers (page 136)
- 1 large avocado
- 2 tomatoes, sliced

Variation

Use flaxseed or other raw cracker in place of pizza crackers.

Directions

Make pizza crackers and nut mayo. Slice tomato and avocado.

Spread nut mayo on cracker then top with a slice tomato and/or avocado. May sprinkle pumpkin seed.

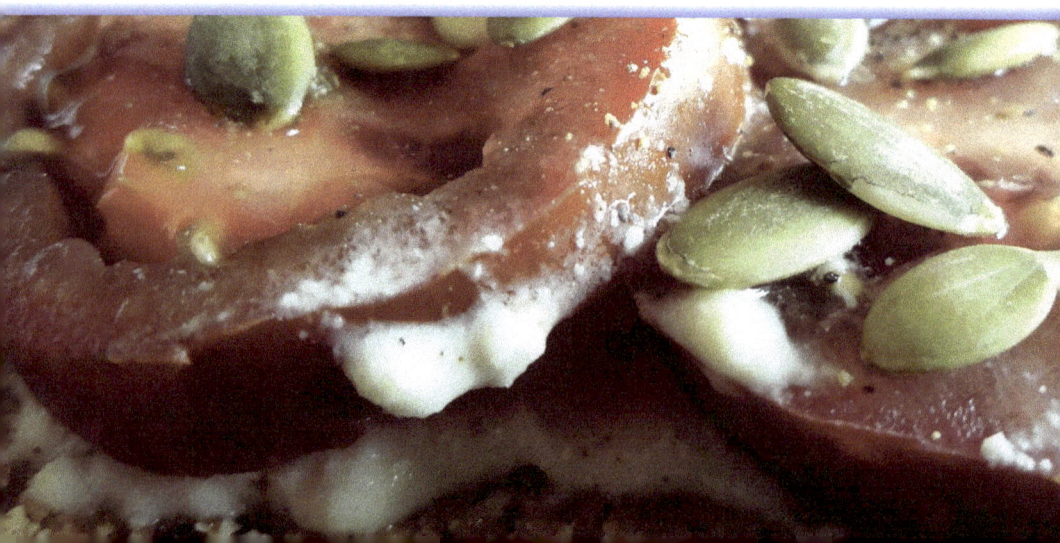

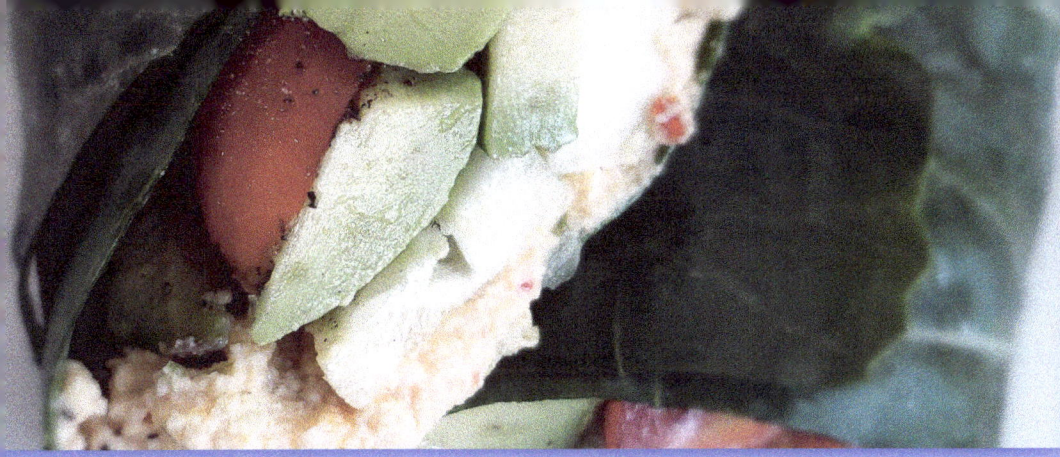

Collard Herb Rolls

Preparation: 30 Min.

Makes 4-6 Servings

Ingredients

- 4-6 large collard green leaves or kale leaves
- 2 c. spicy cheese (page 146)
- 2 small cucumbers, sliced
- 2 avocadoes, sliced
- 2 tomatoes, sliced
- radish and broccoli sprouts

> **Fun Fact**
>
> Collard greens are a form of cabbage.

Directions

Choose largest collard green or kale leaves; wash and dry them with a paper towel. With a sharp knife, remove thick stem from the center of the collard green or kale leaf.

Spread about ½ cup of Spicy Nut Cheese down each spine.

Layer cucumbers, avocado, tomatoes, and sprouts. Roll the leaves and serve.

Eggless Salad Sandwich

Preparation: 30 Min.

Makes 4-6 Servings

Ingredients

- eggless salad (page 34)
- Nancy's bread (page 134)
- green sprouts, such as alfalfa, radish, or sunflower greens.

Variation

Use romaine lettuce in place of bread.

Directions

Prepare eggless salad and Nancy's bread.

Place eggless salad mixture on one slice of bread along with green sprouts. Place another slice of bread on top and enjoy.

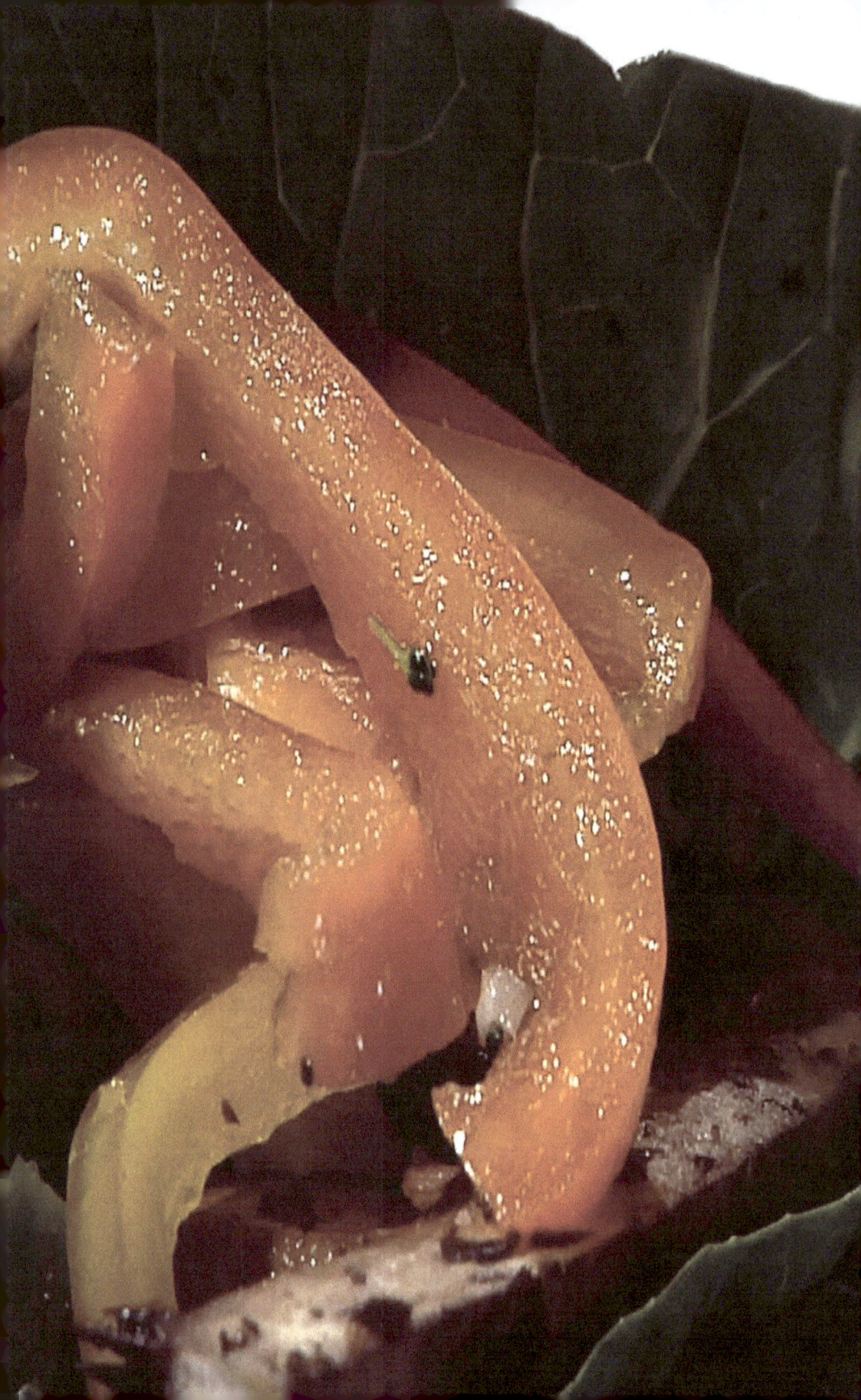

Philly Wrap

Preparation: 10 Min.
Marinating: 30 Min.
Makes 6-8 Servings

Ingredients

- collard greens or cabbage

Mushroom

- 3 Portobello mushrooms, thinly sliced
- ½ c. cold pressed olive oil
- 1 grapefruit, juiced
- 2 tsp. cumin, ground
- 2 tsp. coriander
- 1 tsp. rosemary
- 1 tsp. celery seed
- 1 tbsp. raw apple cider vinegar

Vegetables

- 1 red bell pepper
- 1 yellow bell pepper
- 1 orange bell pepper
- 1 ½ c. broccol
- ½ c. onion
- 1 clove garlic
- 1 tsp. Himalayan crystal salt
- 1 tsp. savory, ground
- ¼ c. cold pressed olive oil

Cheese

- 1 c. sunflower seeds,
- 1 c. pumpkin seeds, soaked
- 3 tbsp. raw apple cider vinegar
- ½ tsp. oregano, dried
- 2 tsp. onion Powder
- 1 tsp. Himalayan crystal salt
- ¼ c. or more water

Directions

Soak sunflower and pumpkin seeds overnight.

'Steak':

Thinly Slice mushrooms and place in a bowl. Juice grapefruit in a small bowl, add oil, vinegar, cumin, coriander, rosemary, and celery seed mix well. Pour over mushrooms making sure they are well coated. Marinate while preparing vegetables.

Vegetables:

Thinly slice red, yellow, and orange bell peppers and place in a dish. Chop broccoli, onion, and garlic place with the peppers. Mix oil, savory, and salt and place over vegetables. Let marinate while preparing the cheese.

Cheese:

Drain the water off sunflower and pumpkin seeds. Place in blender and add vinegar and spice. Blend until smooth adding pure water as needed.

Putting it together:

Wash collard greens or kale; with a knife, remove hard stem keeping the leave as whole as possible. If using cabbage, peel off the large leaves keeping them in one piece.

Lay out green as flat as possible without breaking them. Place the 'steak' on leaf, layer on vegetables and then top with cheese.

Roll or wrap leaf and enjoy the Philly Wrap.

Brazil Nut Burger

Preparation: 20 Min. Soaking: 8-12 Hrs. Drying: 6-12 Hrs. Makes 6-8 Servings

Ingredients

- 2 c. brazil nuts
- ½ c. carrots
- ½ lemon, juiced
- 1 tbsp. garlic powder
- 1 tomatoes
- 1 tbsp. celery seed
- ½ tbsp. poultry seasoning
- ¼ c. dried onion
- ½ c. raw tahini
- 1 tbsp. slippery elm powder
- 1 tbsp. cold pressed olive oil
- Himalayan crystal salt to taste

Directions

Soak Brazil nuts overnight, drain off water, and set aside.

In food processor, combine Brazil nuts, shredded carrots, tomatoes, lemon juice, tahini, garlic, olive oil, and spices until mixed thoroughly.

Shape into burgers and dehydrate on nonstick dehydrator sheets for 2-4 hours. Flip and carefully remove the nonstick dehydrator sheet. Continue drying for another 2-4 hours.

Place on lettuce leaf or cabbage leaf and top with green spouts, avocados and tomatoes.

Fun Fact

One Brazil nut provides 100% of your selenium daily requirement.

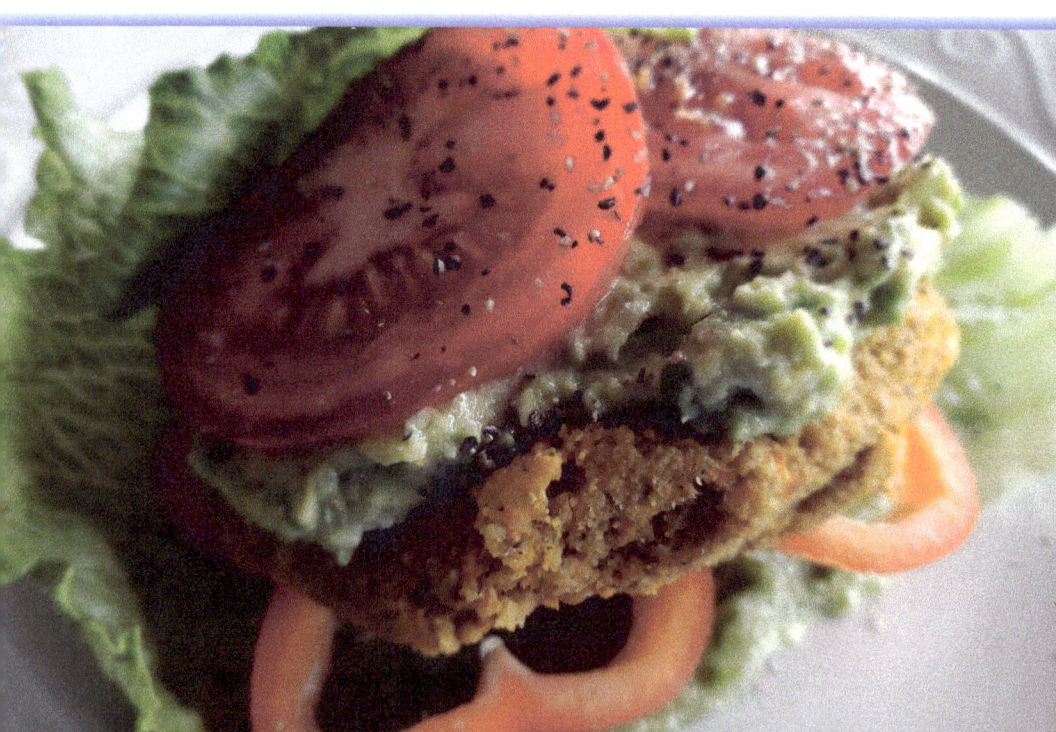

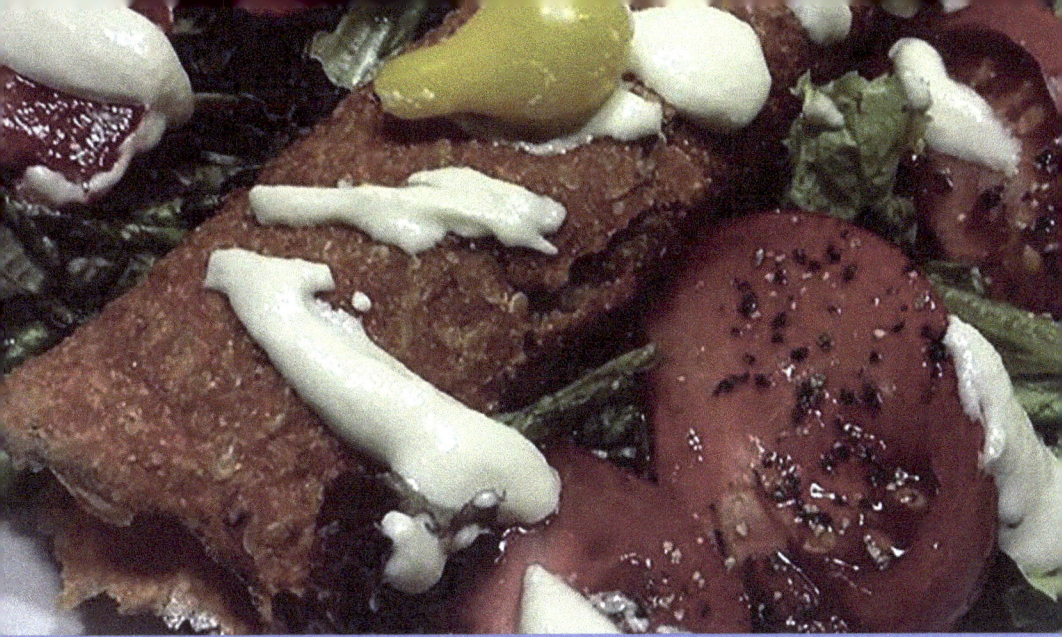

Bean Burrito

Preparation: 30 Min.　　*Soaking:* 20 Min.　　*Drying:* 4-10 Hrs.　　*Makes 6-8 Servings*

Ingredients

Crust

- 1 ½ c. dried tomatoes
- 1 clove garlic
- 2 tsp. Himalayan crystal salt
- ½ c. flax, ground in a coffee grinder
- ¼ onion, chopped
- 1 small hot pepper, seeded and chopped

Filling

- sunflower beans (page 56)
- sour cream (page 144)
- garnish: avocados, tomatoes, sprouts, lettuce

Variation

Instead of making the crust, try using a collard green leaf. Very carefully cut the stem with a knife until it is thin and the leaf is whole.

Directions

Soak dried tomatoes in water for about 20 minutes. Take tomatoes out of water, using water as needed later.

In food processor, mix dried tomatoes, garlic, salt, ground flax seed, onion hot pepper until it looks like dough.

Spread on dehydrator nonstick dehydrator sheets and dry for about 2-4 hours. Turn crust over, spread sunflower beans and roll. Continue drying about 2-6 hours until desired texture is achieved.

Serve on lettuce with tomatoes and avocadoes. Drizzle sour cream over top.

Lasagna

Preparation: 35 Min.
Soaking: 8-12 Hrs.
Drying: 5-10 Hrs.
Makes 6-8 Servings

Ingredients

- 2 tbsp. pumpkin seeds
- ground meatless (page 57)

Zoodles

- 3 large zucchinis

Cheese Sauce

- 2 c. cashews
- 1 clove garlic
- 1 tsp. Italian seasoning
- ½ tsp. Himalayan crystal salt
- 4 tbsp. cold pressed olive oil
- 1 c. pure water as needed

Marinara Sauce

- 1 c. dried tomatoes
- 2-3 c. tomatoes
- 1 tsp. basil
- 1 tsp. oregano
- 1 tsp. Himalayan crystal salt
- 1 clove garlic
- ¼ c. onion

Veggies

- 1 ½ c. spinach, stems removed
- 1 colored bell pepper,
- any other vegetables as desired

Directions

Soak pumpkin seeds. drain water off then roughly chop pumpkin seeds and set aside. Make meatless and marinara sauce.

Zoodles:

Using a mandolin, slice the zucchini into thin slices. Lay them flat on dehydrator tray. Dry at 100° F. for about an hour. These become your zoodles (noodles).

Cheese Sauce:

Place cashews nuts in a blender, add garlic, seasoning and olive oil then mix. Add water in small amounts until a thick smooth texture is reached.

Marinara Sauce:

Soak dried tomatoes in water for 30 minutes.

Place soaked dried tomatoes with the oil in a blender, fresh tomatoes, onion basil, oregano, clove, garlic, and salt mix until smooth.

Vegetables:

Washing spinach and removing stems. Chop colored bell peppers. You can use yellow, red, or orange bell pepper or combination of them. Make deluxe by adding other vegetables.

Putting it all Together:

Place a third of marinara sauce on bottom of a 9x9 pan. Add half of the meatless on top. Using a spoon mix the meatless and marinara. Spread it until it is even.

Layer half of zoodles over the top of the meatless layer.

Evenly spread half the cheese sauce over zoodles. Evenly spread vegetables over cheese sauce. Mix ½ of the remaining marinara with remaining meatless and layer over vegetables. Layer the remaining zoodles over meatless.

Spread cheese sauce over zoodles. Evenly spread remaining marinara over the top and sprinkle pumpkin seeds. Place in a dehydrator at 100° for about 4 hours or until warm.

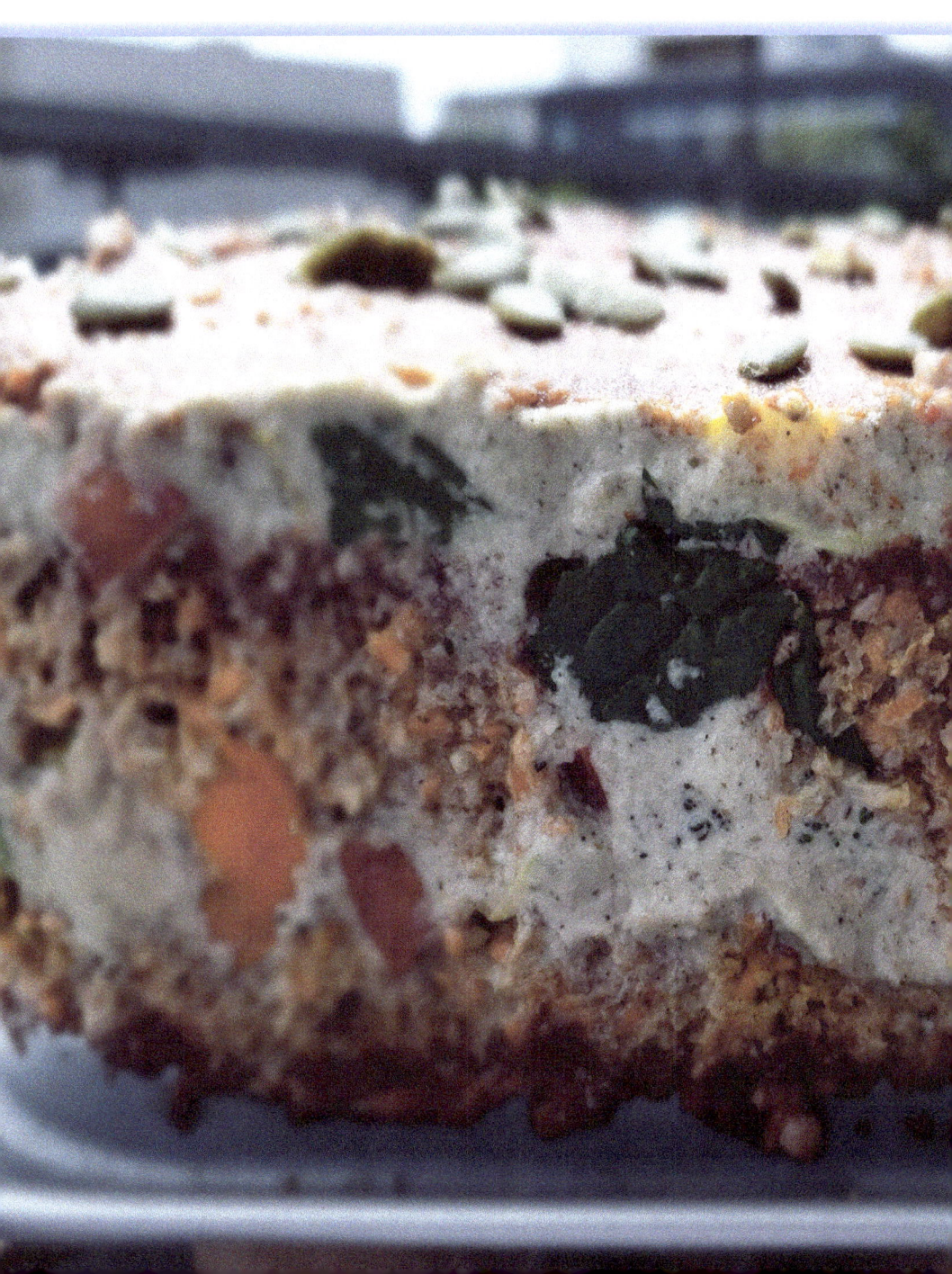

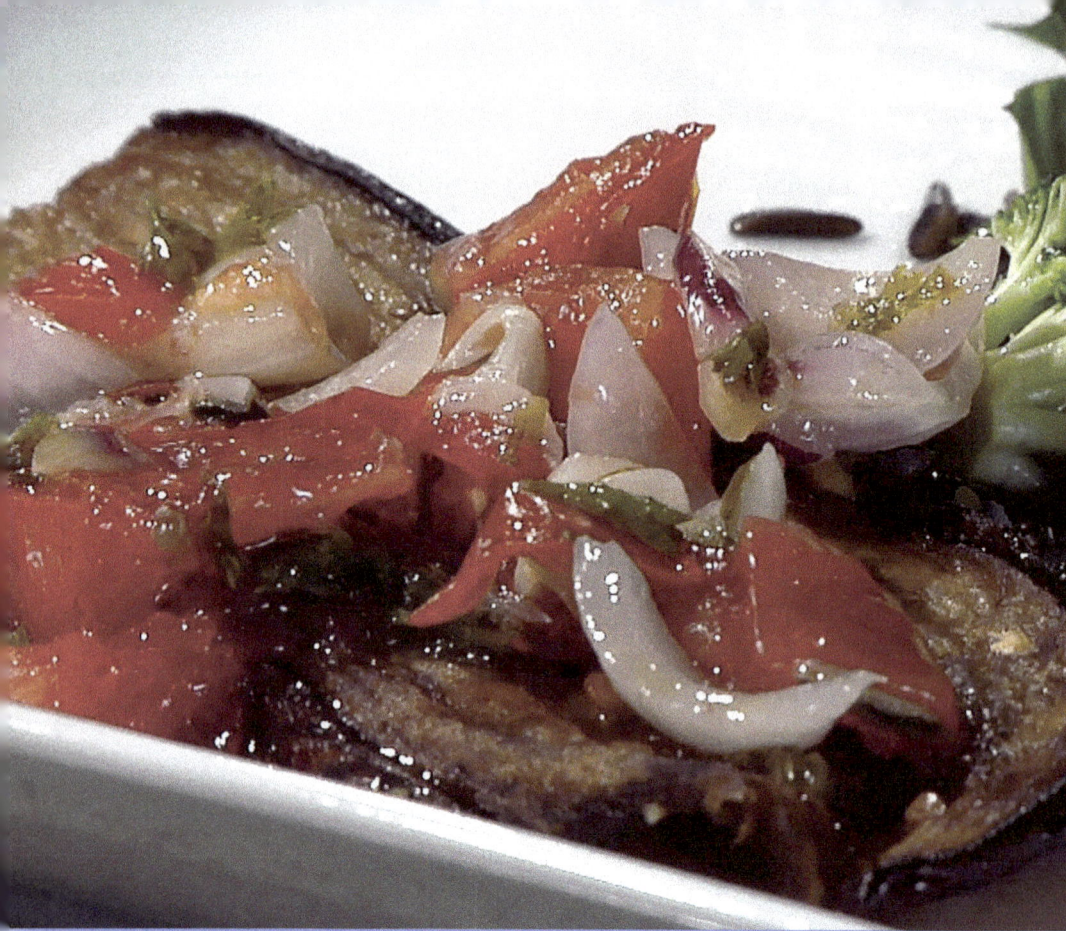

Middle Eastern Marinated Eggplant

Preparation: 10 Min. Chilling: 1-2 Hrs. Makes 6-8 Servings

Ingredients

- 1 ¼ c. cold pressed olive oil
- ½ onion, thinly sliced
- 3 medium tomatoes, chopped
- 2 tbsp. parsley
- 2 tbsp. basil
- 2 eggplants
- 1 lemon, juiced
- Himalayan crystal salt
- lemon wedges to garnish

Directions

Cut eggplants lengthwise into 2-inch-thick stakes. Place oil, onions, lemon juice, parsley, salt, and basil with eggplant. Make sure eggplant is well coated add water if necessary to cover the top and let marinate overnight.

Place in dehydrator for about 7 hours and serve immediately when removed. Garnish with lemon wedges.

Cravin' Mac & Cheese

Preparation: 20 Min.　　Soaking: 8-12 Hrs.　　Drying: 16-18 Hrs.　　Makes 6-8 Servings

Ingredients

Sauce

- ¾ c. cashews
- ¼ c. almonds
- ¼ c. walnuts
- 1 lemon, juiced
- ½ orange, juiced
- ½ tsp. raw apple cider vinegar
- ¾ tsp. Himalayan crystal salt
- 1-2 cloves garlic
- ½ c. cold pressed olive oil
- ¼ tsp. mustard powder
- ¼ c. fresh parsley or 2 tbsp. dried
- ¼ c. pure water

Noodles

- 2 c. butternut squash,
- 2 c. spaghetti squash,

Directions

Soak almonds and walnuts overnight, drain water off, and set nuts aside.

In a blender, combine cashews, almonds, and walnuts along with lemonj uice, orange juice, vinegar, garlic, oil and spice until creamy. Use only enough water to make it a nice creamy consistency.

Use very ripe butternut and spaghetti squash. The riper they are, the easier they are to shred and eat. Cut and shred 2 cups of each squash.

Place shredded squash in a bowl and mix in creamy sauce. May put in dehydrator at 100°F until warm.

Variation

May use zoodles in place of other squash

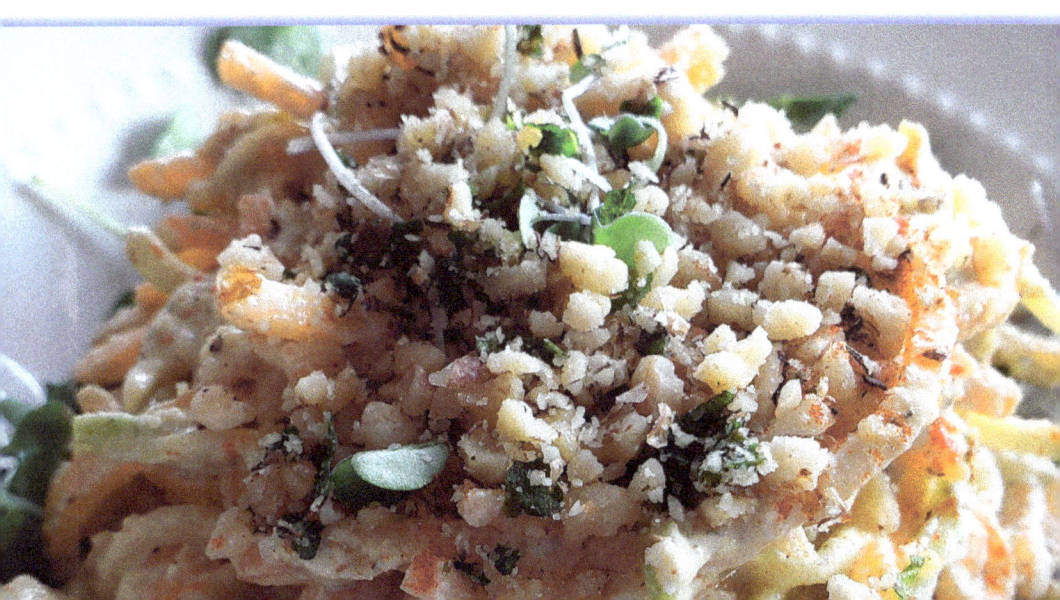

Anytime Breakfast Burrito

Preparation: 20 Min. *Soaking:* 20 Min. *Drying:* 2-4 Hrs. Makes 4-6 Servings

Ingredients

Crust

- 1 ½ c. tomatoes
- 1 clove garlic
- 2 tsp. Himalayan crystal salt
- ½ c. flax, ground in a coffee grinder
- ¼ onion, chopped
- 1 small hot pepper, seeded and chopped

Filling

- eggless salad (page 34)
- garnish:
  sour cream (page 144),
  baykon (page 87),
  avocadoes, tomatoes,
  sprouts, lettuce

Note

Use dried tomatoes; just soak them for 30 minutes before using.

Variation

Use chard leaf or colored green with thick stems cut out for wrap instead of crust.

Directions

In coffee grinder, grind the whole flaxseed. You now have flax meal.

In a food processor, mix garlic, salt, flax meal, onion, hot pepper, and tomatoes, which have been drained. Mix until it looks like a dough. If more moisture is needed, use water tomatoes were soaked in.

Spread dough on dehydrator nonstick dehydrator sheets and dry for about 2-4 hours. Turn crust over, carefully peel off the nonstick dehydrator sheet. Spread with eggless salad and roll.

Continue drying for about 2-6 hours until desired texture is achieved. Serve on lettuce surrounded with tomatoes, avocadoes and baykon. Drizzle sour cream over the top.

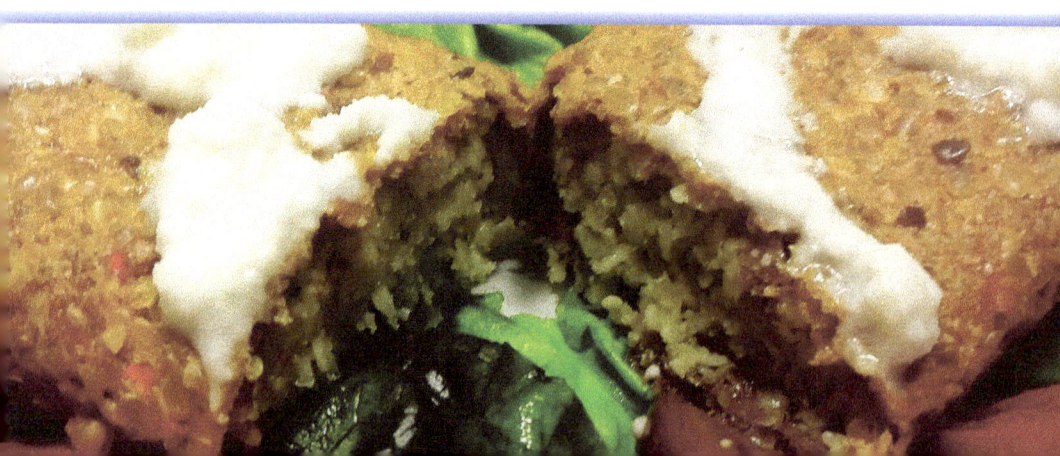

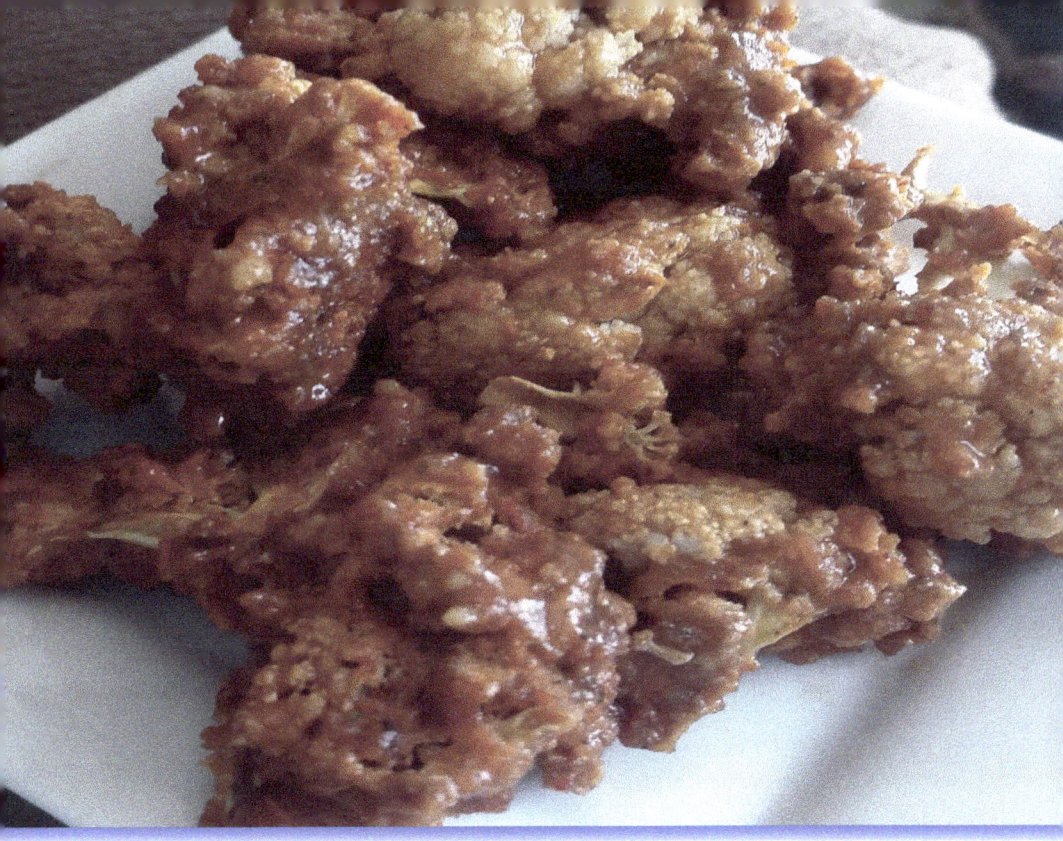

Cauliflower Wings

Preparation: 20 Min. *Marinating:* 2-12 Hrs. *Drying* 4-7 Hrs *Makes 6-8 Servings*

Ingredients

- head of cauliflower
- ½ c. dried tomato
- 1 small fresh tomato
- 1 clove garlic
- 2 tsp. paprika
- 2 tbsp. raw coconut flour
- 1 tsp. dried parsley
- ¾ c. Brother John's tabasco (page 150) or other barbecue sauce

Directions

Soak almonds overnight, drain water off and set aside. Cut 1 head of cauliflower into about 2 inch pieces and set aside.

In a blender, combine tomato, garlic, paprika, coconut flower, and parsley until a thick smooth paste is achieved, adding up to a cup of water if needed.

Toss cauliflower with blender mix, make sure it is well covered. Let sit for 2 hours, I left it overnight.

Place on a dehydrator tray in a single layer and dry about 6 hours. Gently toss with favorite raw or fermented barbecue sauce or hot sauce.

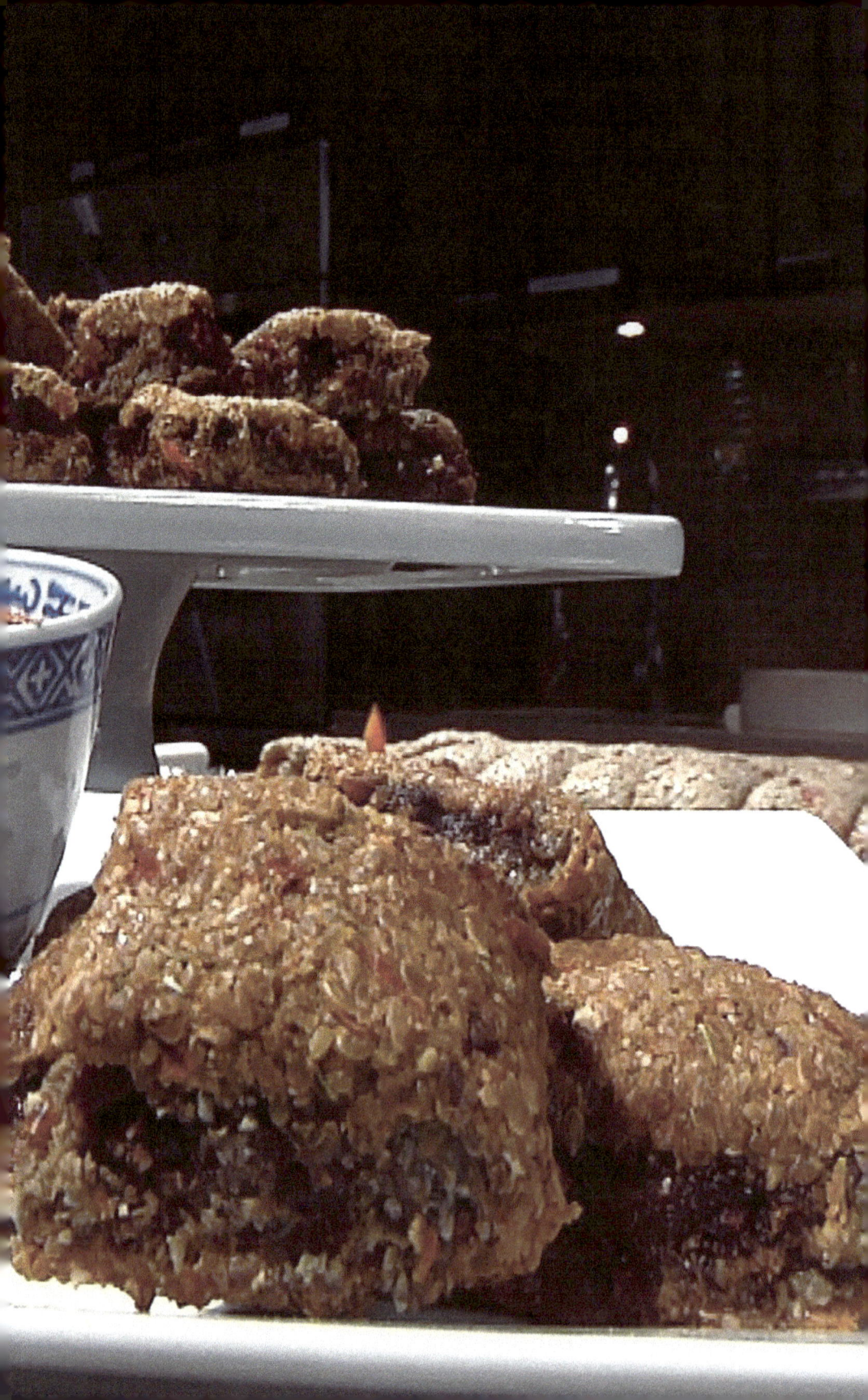

Pizza Bites

| Preparation: | Soaking: | Drying: | Makes 6-8 |
| 35 Min. | 8-12 Hrs. | 5-10 Hrs. | Servings |

Ingredients

Crust

- 1 large onion
- 2-3 stalks of celery
- 3 small tomatoes
- 2-3 cloves of garlic
- 1 tsp. Himalayan crystal salt
- 2 c. golden flax, ground in coffee grinder
- water if needed

Filling

- 1 c. sunflower seeds, soaked
- 1 medium onion
- 1 tbsp. cold pressed olive oil
- 2 tbsp. poultry seasoning
- Himalayan crystal salt

Sauce

- 4 medium tomatoes
- ½ c. dried tomatoes, soaked
- 1 tsp. cold pressed olive oil
- 1 tbsp. pizza seasonings

Toppings

- red bell peppers
- olives
- mushrooms
- whatever else you may enjoy on pizza.

Directions

Crust:

Place chopped onion, celery, tomatoes, garlic, and salt in food processor and mix well. Slowly add flax seed that was ground in a coffee grinder. It should be doughy and dry enough to spread. Spread on nonstick dehydrator sheet about 4 inches wide and about ½ inch thick and set aside. More than one nonstick dehydrator sheet maybe needed.

Filling:

Mix sunflower seeds, onion, olive oil, poultry seasoning, and salt in a food processor, until well mixed then spread over crust.

Sauce:

In blender, mix fresh tomatoes, dried tomatoes, olive oil and pizza seasoning blend until smooth and spread over filling.

Spread chopped toppings over the sauce. Fold one side of the crust to the middle and then the other side to the middle. There is now a seam down the middle. Slice the middle then cut into about 2-inch pieces and dehydrate for about 5-10 hours at a 100 degrees F. It is done when it looks "cooked."

Fun Fact

Hippocrates wrote about using flax for the relief of abdominal pains, and Theophrastus recommend the use of flax mucilage as a cough remedy

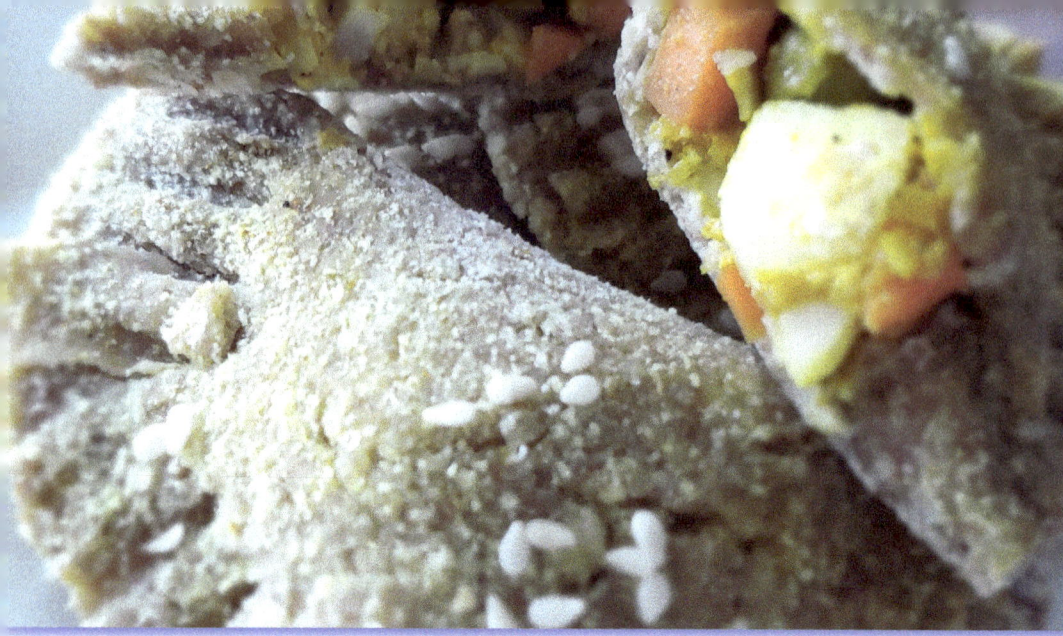

Vegetable Pocket (Samosa)

Preparation: 20 Min.

Makes 4-6 Servings

Ingredients

Crust

- Nancy's bread (page 134)

Filling

- 1 c. turnip
- 1 c. carrot
- 1 c. peas, dried or fresh
- ¼ c. pure water
- 2 tbsp. lemon juice
- 1 tsp. onion powder
- 1 tsp. cumin
- ½ tsp. turmeric
- ¼ tsp. black pepper
- 1 tsp. Himalayan crystal salt

Fun Fact

The WW1 German famine 1916-1917 was known as "turnip winter"

Directions

Chop turnips and carrots, place them in a bowl add peas and set aside.

In a blender, place cashews or almonds, olive oil, water, lemon, juice, onion powder turmeric, cumin pepper and salt and mix until well blended. Pour blended ingredients over vegetables and mix. Set aside and let marinate while making Nancy's bread.

Shape bread into rounds. Place one round on dehydrator tray. Place a spoonful of filling on half of it, fold other half over, and seal it with a fork along the edges (an empanada or dumpling press works well). Repeat until all rounds have been filled. Dehydrate at 100°F for 3 to 6 hours.

Purple Ribbon

Preparation: 35 Min. Marinating: 1-2 Hrs. Makes 6-8 Servings

Ingredients

- 2 c. mushrooms
- 1 c. onion
- 1-2 tsp. parsley
- ¼ lemon, juiced
- 1 tbsp. cold pressed olive oil
- 2 c. sauerkraut, made with red cabbage (page 60)
- ½ c. basic cheese (page 145)
- rye bread (page 133)

Directions

Make basic cheese, sauerkraut and rye bread set aside.

Marinate thinly sliced onions and mushrooms, with parsley in olive oil and lemon juice for 30 minutes. Stir in cheese and place on one slice of rye bread place the purple sauerkraut on top. Cover with a second slice of rye and serve.

Fun Fact

This is my answer to a Reuben sandwich. The mushrooms make wonderful substitute for meat, topped off with red sauerkraut and served on raw rye bread.

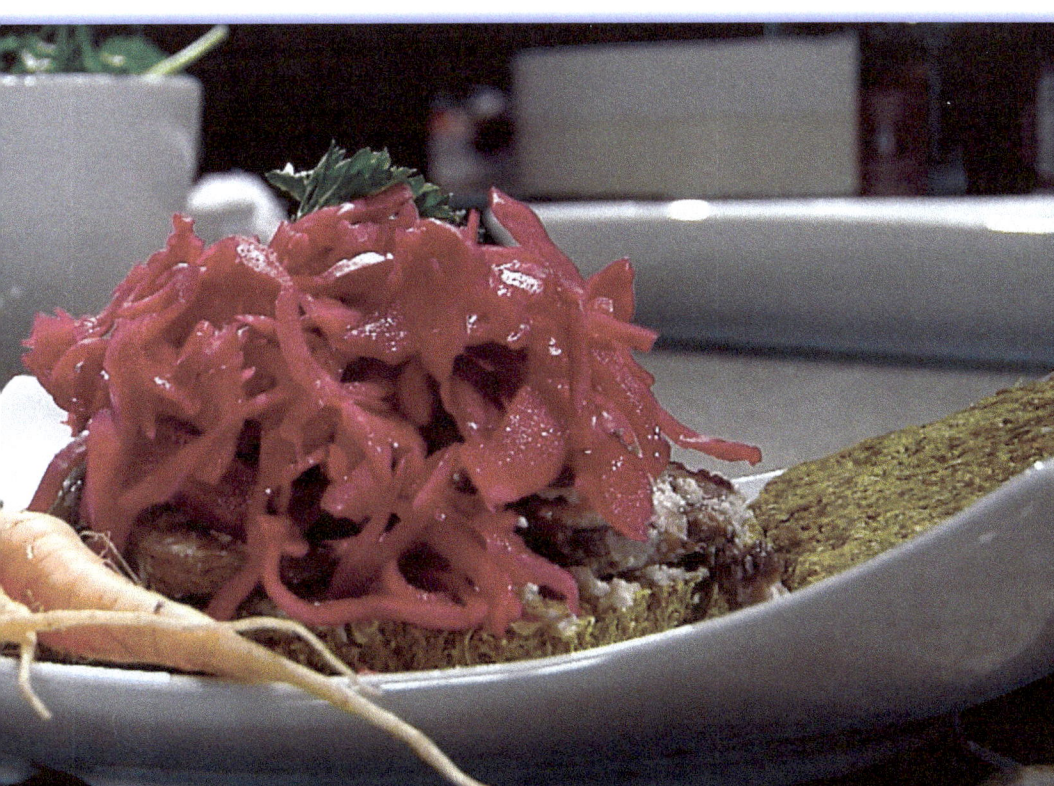

Almond Delight

Preparation: 30 Min.

Makes 4-6 Servings

Ingredients

Pepper Sauce

- 1 c. almonds
- 1 red bell peppers
- ½ tsp. dried thyme
- ½ tsp. dried tarragon
- ½ tsp. dried marjoram
- pinch paprika
- ¼ tsp. Himalayan crystal salt
- ¼ c. pure water (more or less as needed)

"Pasta"

- 3-4 small zucchinis
- 1 c. broccoli
- ½ c. asparagus
- 3 large yellow or red bell peppers
- 2 c. spinach, chopped
- ½ c. fresh basil, chopped
- 2 tsp. poppy seeds
- Himalayan crystal salt
- pepper to taste

Directions

Soak almonds overnight. Peel the brown skin off wet almonds and drain the water.

Mix almonds, chopped bell pepper, thyme, tarragon, marjoram, paprika, salt, and water in a blender until smooth and creamy. (More or less water may be needed.)

Shred zucchini and asparagus. Chop broccoli, bell pepper, spinach, basil, add to bowl with zucchini and asparagus along with poppy seeds, salt, and pepper then place in a bowl.

Gently toss together pepper sauce with the vegetable "pasta." Garnish with tomatoes.

Fun Fact

Almonds are members of the rose family.

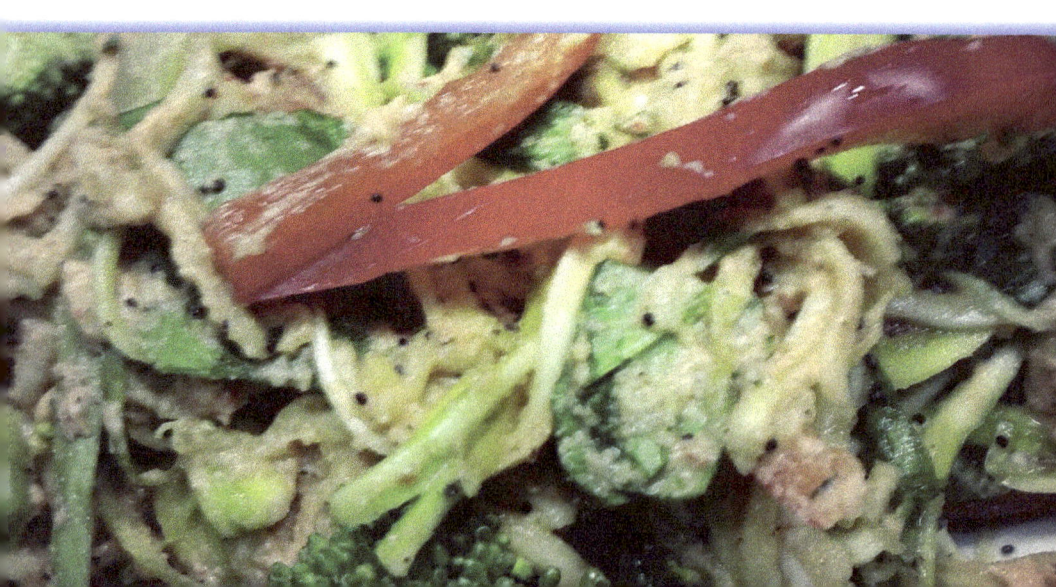

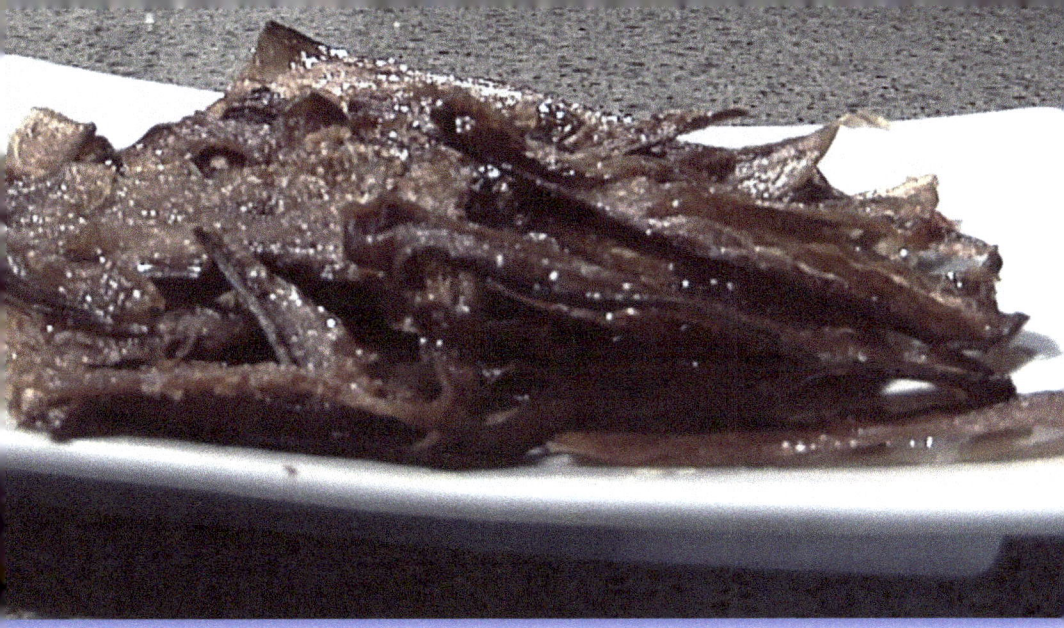

Baykon

Preparation: 15 Min. **Marinating:** 2-24 Hrs **Drying:** 12-18 Hrs. **Makes 6-8 Servings**

Ingredients

- 2 large Asian eggplants
- ¼ - ½ c. cold pressed olive oil
- 2 tbsp. raw apple cider vinegar
- 1 grapefruit, juiced
- 3 tbsp. Himalayan crystal salt

Directions

Cut off top and bottom of eggplant. While any kind of eggplant will work, Asian eggplant, the long thin one, will look more like bacon.

Using a mandolin, thinly slice eggplant lengthwise. It should be long strips of thin eggplant.

Layer sliced eggplant on bottom of marinating pan. Sprinkle some salt over top. Add another layer of sliced eggplant, add more salt, and continue until eggplant is all laid out.

Pour olive oil over top of eggplant, add vinegar and grapefruit juice. If eggplant is not covered, use a little bit of water.

Marinate at least 2 hours and up to 24 hours. The eggplant may darken. That is okay; it is just oxidation.

Using dehydrator trays, place marinated baykon out to dry in single layers.

Dehydrate about 18 hours. Baykon should be crispy when done

Note

For easy clean up, place a nonstick dehydrator sheet on the bottom of dehydrator to catch the dripping oil.

Shepherd's Pie

Preparation: 20 Min. | Sprouting: 1-5 Days | Marinating: 20 Min. | Drying: 3-6 Hrs. | Makes 2-4 Servings

Ingredients

Gravy

- ½ c. dried tomatoes
- ¼ c. onion, chopped
- ½ red bell pepper, chopped
- 1 clove garlic
- 1 tsp. basil
- ½ tsp. cumin seed, ground
- ½ tsp. oregano
- 1 tsp. Himalayan crystal salt

Hash

- ½ c. corn
- ½ c. mixed sprouts, sprouted 1-5 days
- ½ red bell pepper, sliced
- ½ orange bell pepper, sliced
- ½ yellow bell pepper, sliced
- ½ c. tomatoes, chopped
- ½ tsp. Italian seasoning
- 1 tsp. turmeric
- ½ tsp. black pepper

Topping

- ½ c. turnip, peeled and chopped
- ½ c. rutabaga, peeled and chopped
- 1 c. parsnip, peeled and chopped
- 2 tsp. cold pressed olive oil
- 1 lime, juiced
- ¼ c. onion, chopped
- 1 tsp. Himalayan crystal salt
- 1 clove garlic
- black pepper to taste

Directions

Sprout bean mix, any combination of adzuki beans, green peas, mung beans, fenugreek.

Gravy

Soak dried tomatoes for about 20 minutes soaked in enough water to cover. Drain water from tomatoes and place in blender. Add onion, ½ red bell pepper, garlic clove, basil, cumin, oregano, salt, and pepper blend until well mixed. Add tomato water if too thick.

Hash

In a bowl, mix corn kernel, sprouts, chopped tomatoes, bell peppers, oregano, turmeric, and black pepper. Combine tomato mixture and stir by hand. Place on the bottom of 2-quart pan.

Topping

Peel and chop turnip, parsnip, and rutabaga and place in a food processor or blender, combine with olive oil, lime juice, onion, garlic, salt, and pepper, mix until mashed texture is achieved Spread turnip topping over top of mixture in pan. Sprinkle with paprika if desired. Dehydrate about 4 hours a 100°F.

Note

May replace rutabaga with turnip or white carrot.

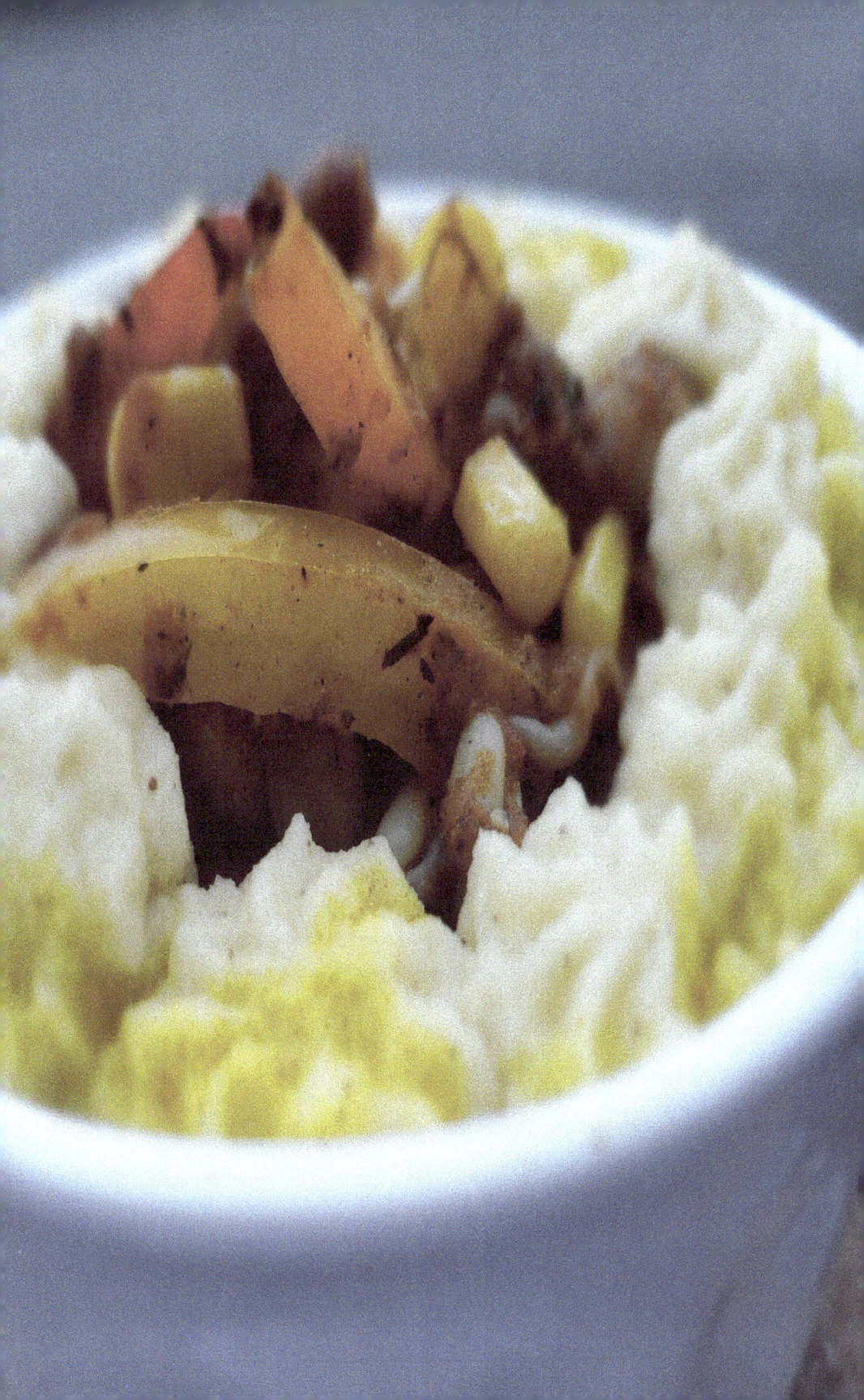

Baja Pulled Eggplant Burrito

Preparation: 15 Min. Marinating: 2-24 Hrs Drying: 18-24 Hrs. Makes 4-6 Servings

Ingredients

- coconut wraps**

Pulled Eggplant

- 2 large Japanese eggplants
- ½ to 1 cup olive oil
- 1 ½ tbsp. taco seasoning
- 2 ½ tsp. Himalayan crystal salt
- 1 tbsp. poultry seasoning

Burrito Stuffing

- 1 ear of corn
- 1 ½ cups sprouted black beans*
- 1 large tomato
- ¼ cup onion
- 1 avocado

Baja Sauce

- ½ c. nut mayo (page 143)
- 1 lime, juiced
- 1 ½ tsp. taco seasoning
- 1 tsp. ground cumin
- small amount of salt
- pepper to taste

Directions

Pulled Eggplant

Julienne, or cut eggplant into long thin strips, marinate overnight, or longer if desired, in olive oil, salt, and taco seasoning. Place strips on dehydrator mesh and dry until it has a meaty texture, about 8-10 hours.

Black Bean

Sort and wash the black beans, place into a large glass container, and cover with water. Make sure beans are completely covered; the beans will expand. Soaking at least 8 hours or overnight, rinse them thoroughly or until the water runs clear.

Place beans into a colander, with a plate under, and let them sit and sprout, rinsing them every 8-12 hours. Cover the colander with a towel. The length of time for sprouting will depend on the temperate in your home.

In winter, it usually takes a full 24 hours to see even a tiny sprout; in the summer, it can be as quick as 12 hours. They are ready to steam as soon as you start to see a "tail" or sprout. The beans are steamed to remove bitterness.

Fill steamer pot with as much water as needed and bring to a boil. Place the sprouted beans into the steamer basket, set them over the boiling pot, and cover. Steam the beans for three to four minutes or until tender.

Stuffing

Place sprouted and steamed beans in a large bowl. Chop tomato, avocado, and onion into a bowl. Cut kernels off corncob and place in bowl then gently toss with baja sauce.

Baja Sauce

Place nut mayo in a small bowl with lime juice, taco seasoning, cayenne pepper, cumin and salt and pepper to taste. **Note** the eggplant is salty.

The wrap is a purchased raw coconut wrap. Place a heaping scoop of the mixture from the bowl into the center of coconut wrap then layer pulled eggplant and wrap. Eat immediately or the pulled eggplant will soften.

Notes

*If you want to make a 100% raw, replace the black beans with raw olives.

**Raw coconut wrap can be purchased or made by you.

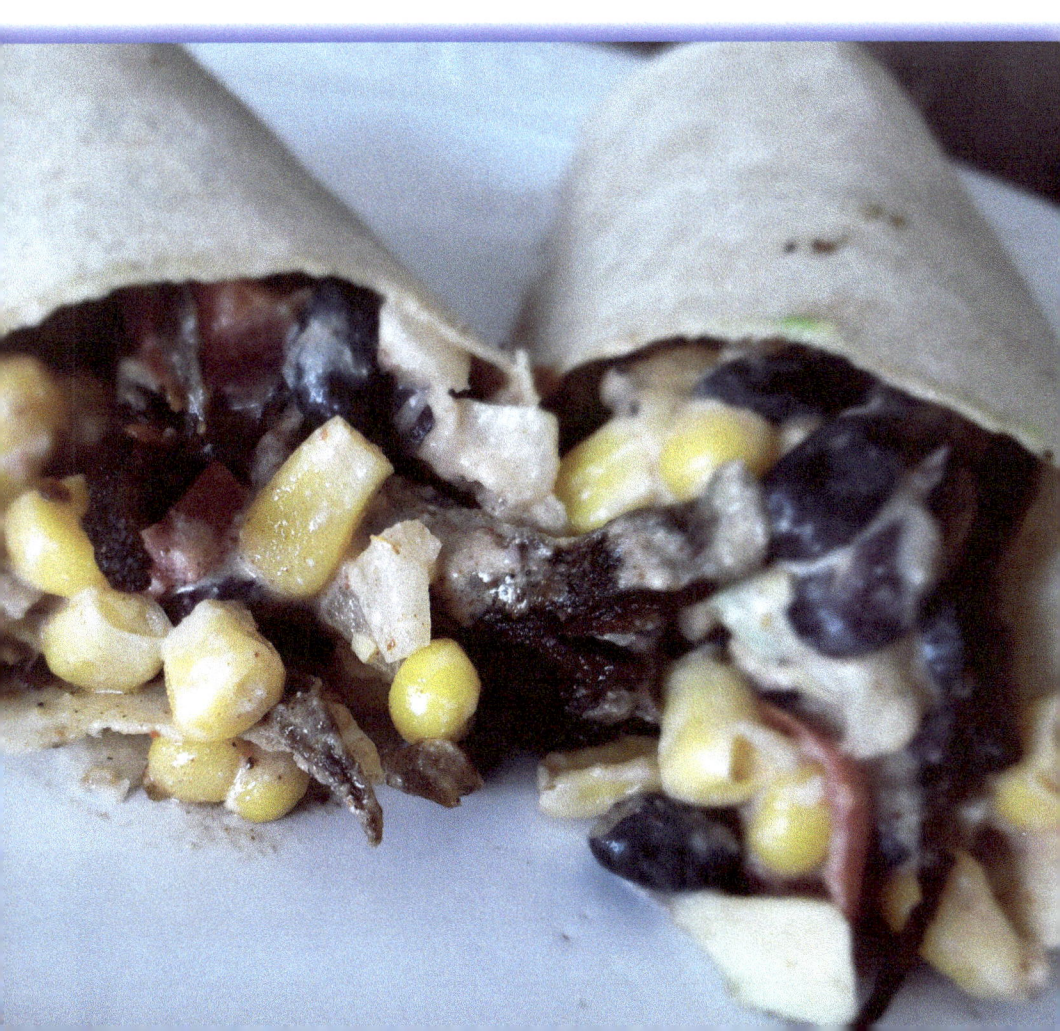

Green Zoodles

Preparation: 20 Min. *Makes 4-6 Servings*

Ingredients

Pesto

- ½ c. fresh spinach leaves
- ¼ c. fresh parsley
- 1 tbsp. dried basil
- 1 tbsp. dried oregano
- 1-3 cloves garlic
- 1-2 green onion
- ½ c. pumpkin seeds
- ½ small zucchini
- 2 or more tsp. cold pressed olive oil
- Himalayan crystal salt to taste
- pure water as needed

Zoodles

- 3-6 small zucchinis

Directions

Soak pumpkin seeds in water at least 3 hours. They can be soaked overnight if desired. Drain water off.

Make pesto by placing spinach, parsley, garlic, onion, zucchini, pumpkin seeds, oil and spices in a food processor or blender. Puree to semi-smooth paste. Add water as needed.

Use a spiral slicer or shred zucchini to look like spaghetti. Place on a plate and pour pesto over top. Garnish with parsley and pumpkin seeds.

Stuffed 'Eggs'

Preparation: 30 Min. *Makes 6-8 Servings*

Ingredients

- ½ c. sesame pulp, saved from milk or soaked sesame seeds
- ½ tsp onion powder
- ½ tsp. parsley
- ½ tsp. dill
- 1 ½ tsp. mustard powder
- 1 tsp. lovage
- ¼ c. nut mayo (page 143)
- Himalayan crystal salt to taste
- pepper to taste
- 8-12 mushrooms caps

Directions

Clean mushrooms and remove stems. Place mushroom caps on a platter stem side up, set aside.

In a bowl mix sesame pulp, onion powder, parsley, dill, mustard powder, lovage and nut mayo. Place sesame mixture inside the mushroom cap.

Variation

Instead of mushrooms use half an avocado

Buttered Zucchini

Preparation: 10 Min. *Makes 6-8 Servings*

Ingredients

Butter Sauce

- ¼ tsp. turmeric
- ½ tsp. Himalayan crystal salt
- ¼ c. cold pressed olive oil, more as desired

Noodles

- 4 c. zucchini
- ¼ c. onion
- ¼ c. sunflower seeds,
- ¼ c. pumpkin seeds,
- 1 tbsp. dried basil
- ½ tsp. black pepper

Directions

Use a spiral slicer or shred zucchini for zoodles and place in a large bowl. Add onion, sunflower, pumpkin seeds, basil and black pepper and gently toss together.

In a small bowl mix oil, turmeric and salt. This is the "butter" sauce. Pour butter sauce over zucchini noodles and gently toss.

Fun Fact
A zucchini has more potassium than a banana.

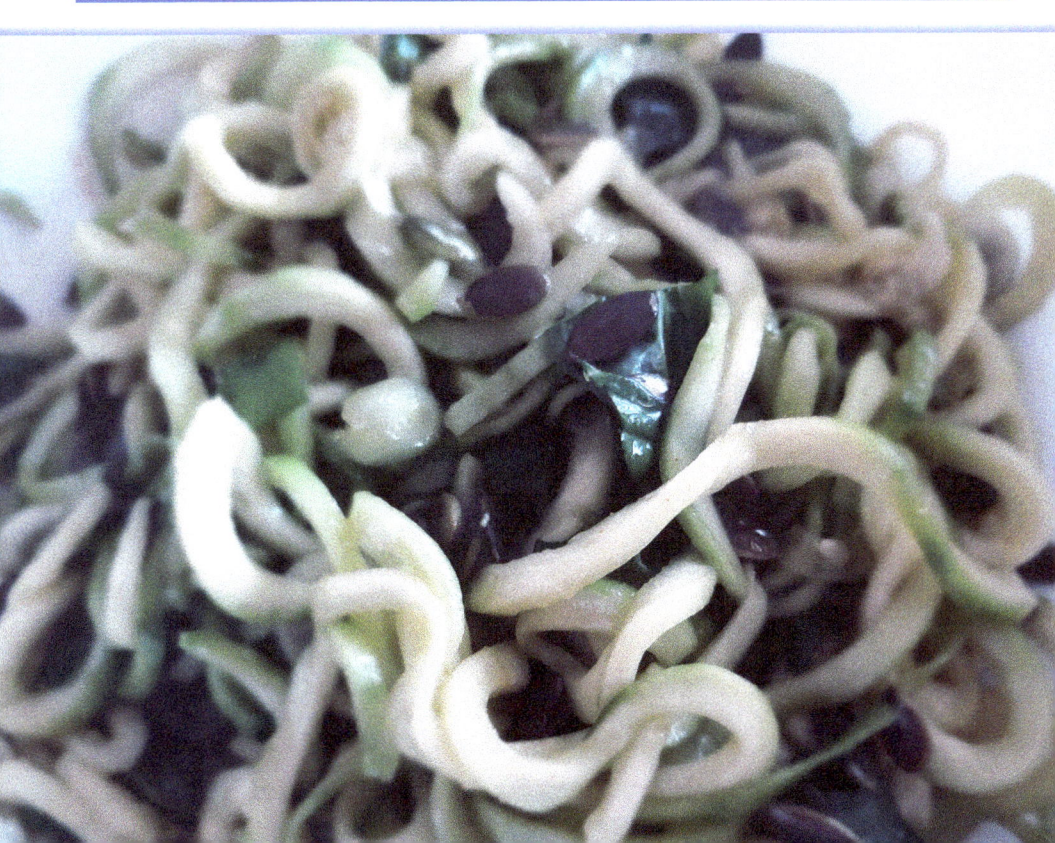

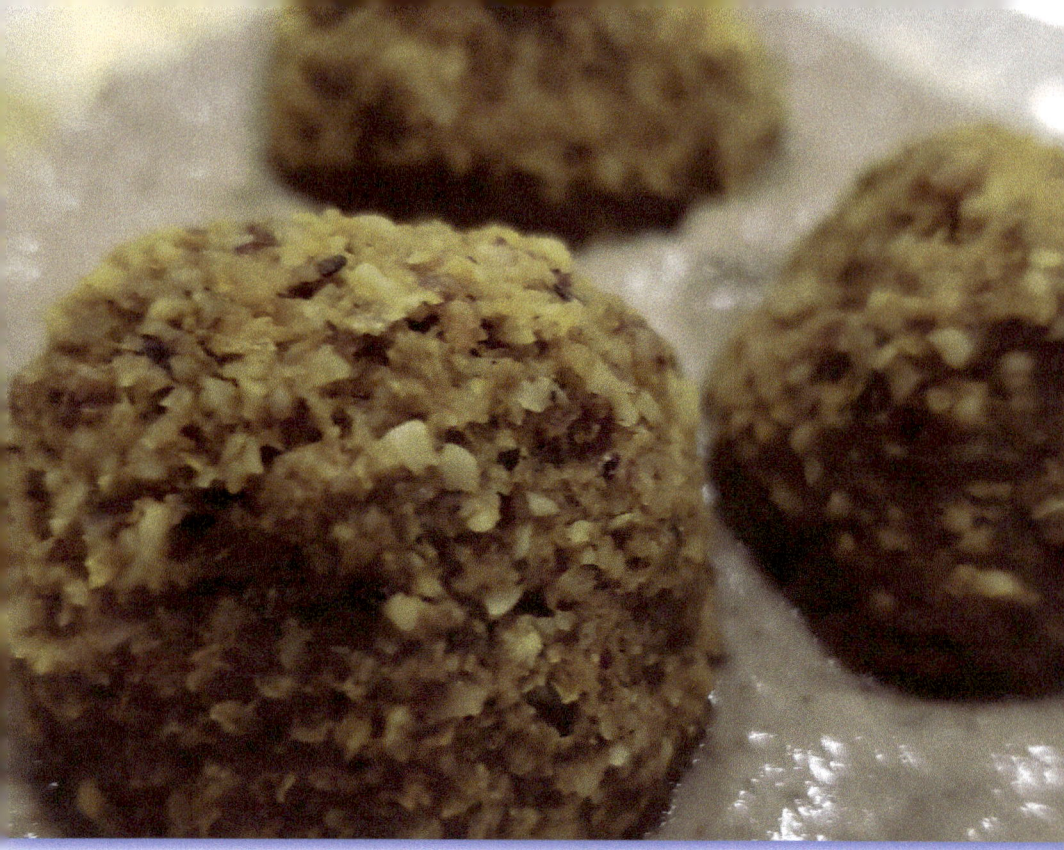

Nutty Pumpkin Balls

| Preparation: | Soaking: | Drying: | Makes 4-6 |
| 35 Min. | 8-12 Hrs | 4-8 Hrs. | Servings |

Ingredients

- ½ c. Brazil nuts
- 1 ½ c. pumpkin
- 3 tbsp. sour cream (page 144)
- 1 tbsp. onion
- ½ c. walnuts
- 1 clove garlic
- 1 ½ tsp. Himalayan crystal salt
- ½ tsp. poultry seasoning
- ¾ tsp. pepper
- ½ tsp. turmeric
- ½ c. red bell pepper
- ¼ c. celery
- 2 tbsp. olive oil
- 1 tbsp. psyllium husk

Directions

Make sour cream and set aside.

Soak Brazil nuts and walnuts overnight. Drain off water and place nuts in a food processor add shredded pumpkin, chopped celery, red bell pepper, onion, garlic, poultry seasoning, pepper, and salt then finely mix. Stir in sour cream by hand.

Form mixture into small balls and place onto dehydrator sheet. Dry 2-8 hours until desired texture is achieved.

Cauliflower Tacos

Preparation: 30 Min. *Marinating:* 1-2 Hrs. *Makes 2-4 Servings*

Ingredients

- 2 c. cauliflower
- 1 c. tomatoes
- 1 garlic, clove
- 1 tsp. cayenne powder
- 1 lime, juiced
- 1 tsp. chili powder
- 2 tsp. cumin
- Himalayan crystal salt to taste
- black pepper to taste
- 1 avocado
- almond sour cream
- romaine lettuce

Directions

Chop cauliflower in food processor until small pieces then place in bowl.

In a blender, combine tomatoes, garlic, cayenne powder, chili powder, cumin, salt, pepper, and lime juice until well mixed.

Pour blender mixture over cauliflower and mix. Let flavors mingle for an hour or more.

Wash and dry romaine lettuce leaf. Fill will cauliflower mixture and top with almond sour cream, sliced avocado and ½ cup chopped tomatoes.

Fun Fact

Mark Twain's wrote "a cauliflower is nothing but a cabbage with a college education."

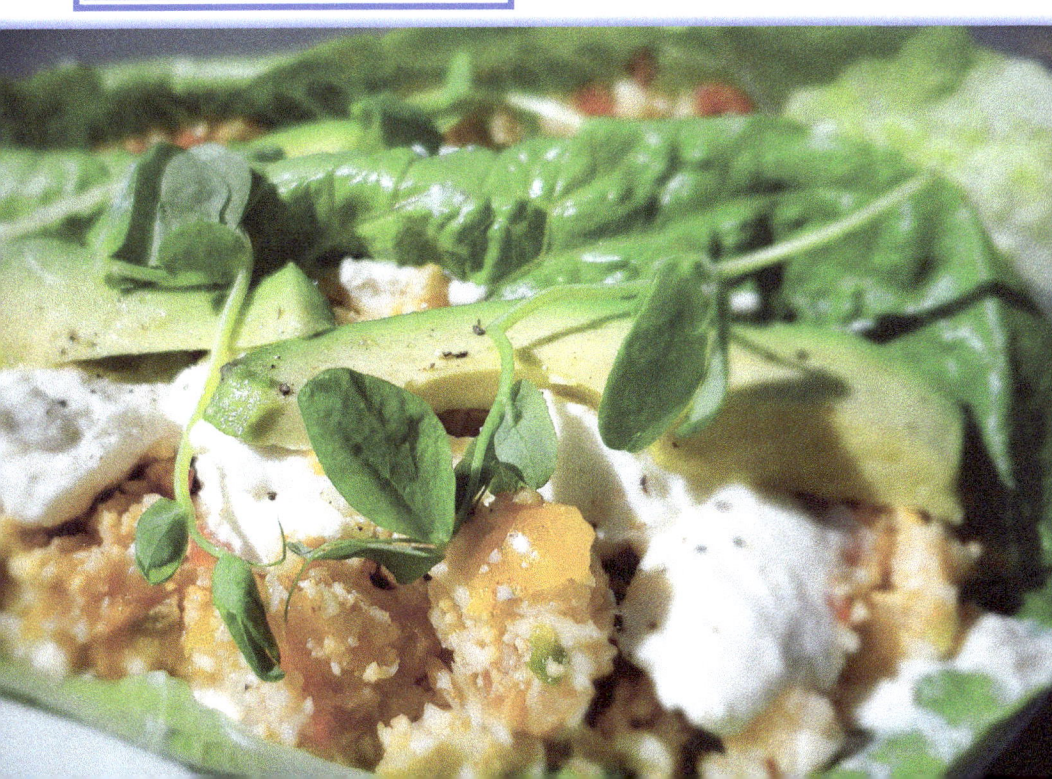

Eggplant Kebabs

Preparation: 30 Min. Marinating: 4-12 Hrs. Drying: 12-14 Hrs. Makes 2-4 Servings

Ingredients

- 1 lime, juiced
- 2 tsp. cumin
- 1 tsp. Himalayan crystal salt
- ¼ tsp. cayenne
- ¾ c. nut mayo (page 143)
- 1 eggplant
- 1 yellow bell pepper
- 1 red bell pepper
- ½ medium onion
- 2 medium zucchinis
- 1 clove garlic
- 1 tbsp. ginger
- ½ tsp. raw apple cider vinegar
- ¼ tsp. turmeric
- ½ tsp. coconut liquid aminos (optional)

Directions

Cut eggplant into 1 inch thick rounds then cut into wedges set aside.

In a blender, place garlic, ginger, lime juice, cumin, salt, nut mayo, turmeric, and cayenne blend until well mixed.

Pour half the marinade over the cut eggplant and let sit for 4-8 hours or longer.

Place marinated eggplant onto a dehydrator try and dry for about 6-7 hours.

Cut onion, yellow and red bell peppers into wedges. Slice the zucchini into rounds place the vegetables in a bowl or jar and remaining marinate for 4-8 hours or longer.

Thread eggplant, bell pepper, onion, and zucchini onto skewers. Place in dehydrator for about 7 hours.

Fun Fact

Some say kebabs can be traced to Turkey where soldiers skewered food on their swords to grill on open fires.

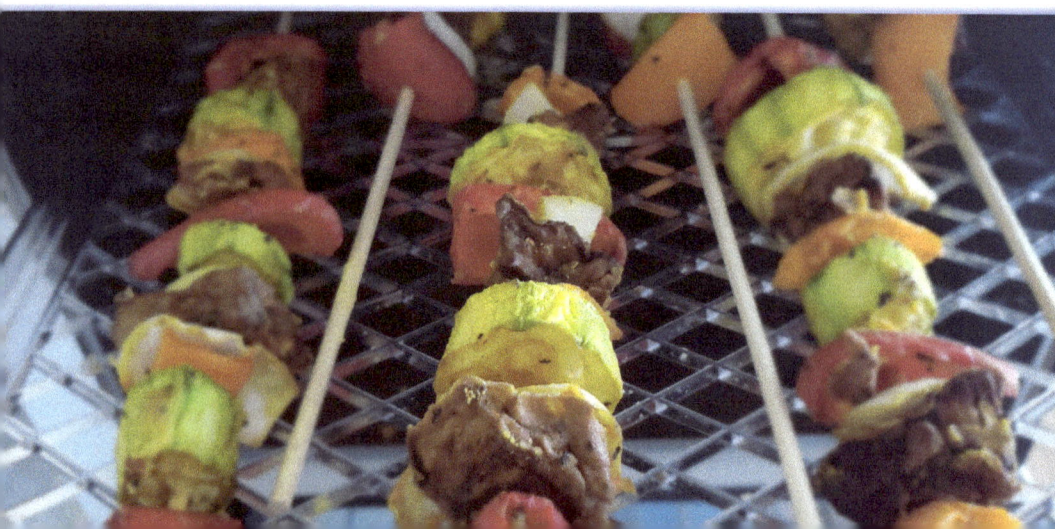

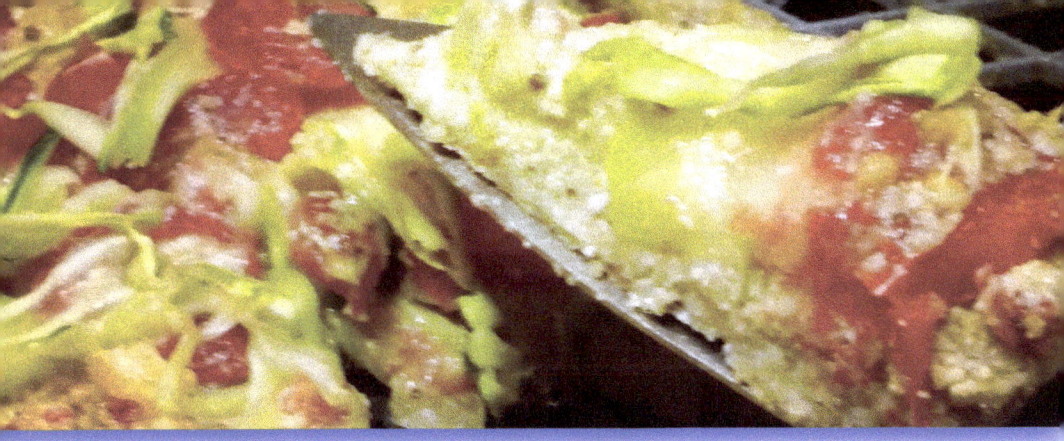

Impossible Zucchini Pie

Preparation: 20 Min.

Makes 4-6 Servings

Ingredients

Crust:

- 1 c. golden flax seed
- 1 c. buckwheat
- 1 tbsp. Himalayan crystal salt
- 1-2 c. pure water
- ¼ c. raw coconut flour (optional)

Filling:

- 1 c. Spicy Nut Cheese (page 146)
- 4 tbsp. cold pressed olive oil
- 3 c. zucchini
- 1 large onion
- ½ red bell pepper
- 1 c. parsley
- 1 carrot
- 2 stocks celery

Directions

Make spicy nut cheese and set aside.

Cover buckwheat with pure water and soak for at least an hour, (may soak overnight if desired), then drain and rinse. Place buckwheat in a food processor.

Grind flax in a coffee grinder. Place flax in food processor with buckwheat and salt, mix using only enough water to make dough.

Roll dough out into a circle on a thin cutting board (this makes it easier to move to the dehydrator tray). Use coconut flour to keep dough from sticking (ground flax seed may be used in place of coconut flour).

Move crust to dehydrator tray. Fold up edges, so crust can hold the filling. Dry about an hour.

Grate zucchini and carrots and place in a bowl. Chop onion and parsley add to zucchini and carrots. Thinly slice bell pepper and celery and mix with the carrots and zucchini. Add spicy nut cheese gently mix all vegetates together.

Place zucchini mixture in the prepared crust and dehydrate at 100° for another 3-5 hours.

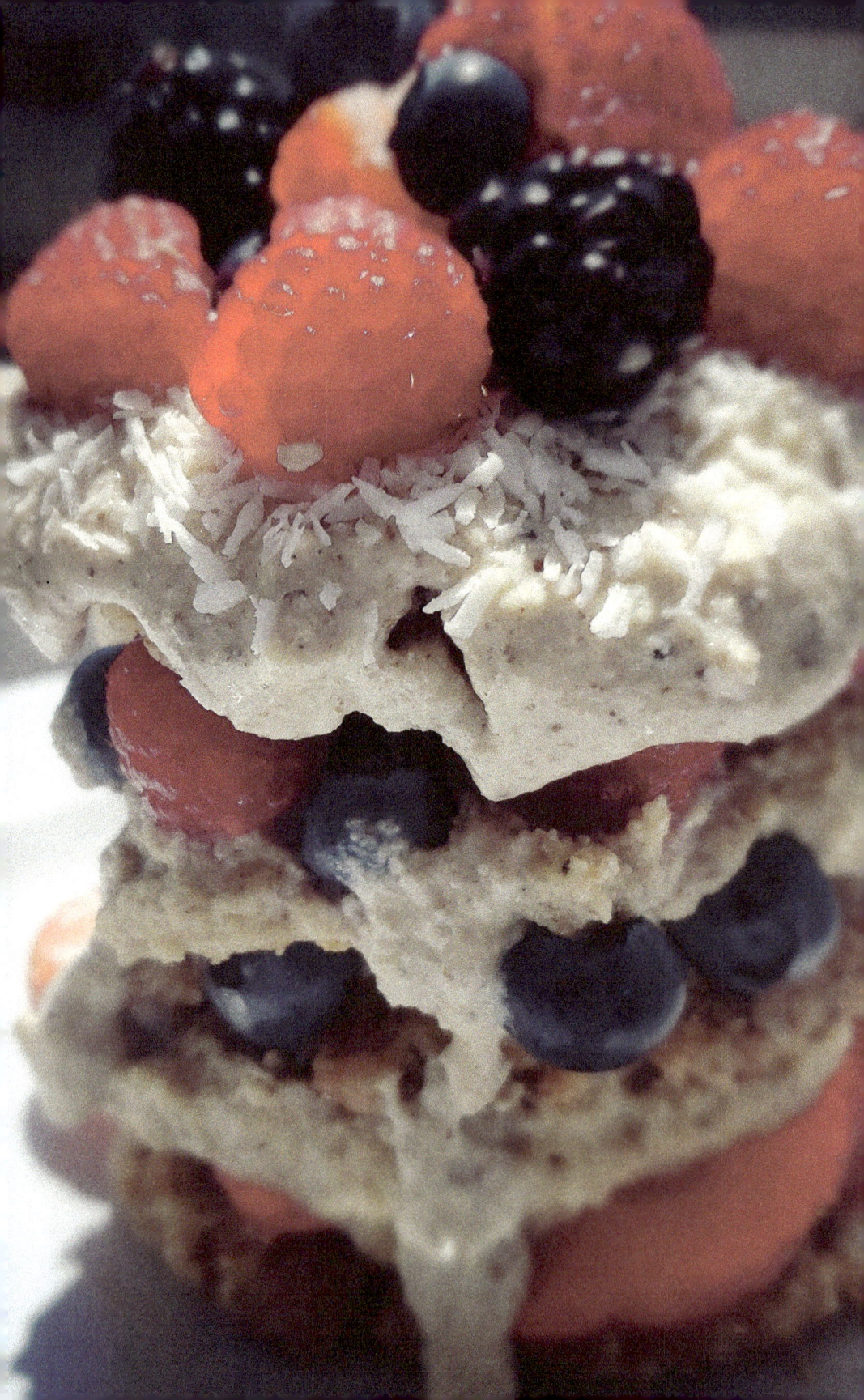

Berry Tall Cake

Preparation: 30 Min. *Drying: 8-12 Hrs.* *Makes 6-8 Servings*

Ingredients

Cake

- 2 c. almonds
- ½ c. dates, pitted
- 1 inch vanilla bean or 1 tsp. vanilla extract

Walnut Cream Topping

- 2 c. walnuts
- ¼ c. raw liquid sweetener
- 1 tbsp. water

Fruit Toppings

- 2 bananas, sliced
- 1 quart berries (any combination)
- shredded coconut

Directions

Soak almonds and walnuts overnight in separate bowls. Drain water off and set aside.

In a food processor, combine almonds, dates and vanilla until well mixed. Form into equal size rounds and set cake aside.

Using a blender make walnut cream by combing soaked walnuts, sweetener and water as need until creamy.

Slice berries and bananas.

Place a cake round on your plate, layer berries and bananas, and then pour walnut cream over top.

Place another cake round on top and repeat until you have only one cake round left on top.

Top with the remaining walnut cream. Cover with coconut and decorate with berries.

Carob Frosting

Preparation: 10 Min. *Makes 6-8 Servings*

Ingredients

- 1 c. raw carob
- ½ c. raw coconut oil
- ½ c. raw liquid sweetener
- ¼ - ¾ c. water

Directions

In a bowl, combine carob, coconut oil, and raw liquid sweetener, until evenly mixed and smooth. Add only enough water until desired thickness and smoothness is achieved.

German Chocolate Donuts

Preparation: 20 Min. Drying: 6-8 Hrs. Makes 6-8 Servings

Ingredients

- 1 ½ c. pecans
- ¾ c. dates
- ½ c. prunes
- ½ c. carob powder
- ¾ c. cacao powder
- 2 tbsp. lemon, juiced
- ¼ c. shredded coconut
- ¼ c. coconut flour

Frosting

- ¾ c. cashews
- ½ c. water
- 1 ½ tbsp. coconut oil
- 2 tbsp. coconut nectar
- ½ tbsp. vanilla
- ¾ c. shredded coconut
- ½ c. pecans, chopped

Variation

For German Chocolate Cake shape the donut dough into cake rounds and dry. Spread the frosting in between each layer.

Directions

Soak dates and prunes for 20 minutes. Save the water for use later.

In a food processor, mix pecans, dates, and prunes until well combined. Add carob, cacao powder, and lemon juice to the nut mixture until well mixed. If too thick add a little water. Mix in coconut flour and shredded coconut by hand.

Shape into donuts or use a donut pan and place in dehydrator for about 2 hours. Remove from the donut pan and continue to dry for another 3-5 hours.

In a blender, mix cashews, date water, coconut oil, coconut nectar and vanilla until smooth. Pour into a bowl. To the bowl stir in the shredded coconut and chopped pecans. Frost the donuts with coconut frosting and enjoy.

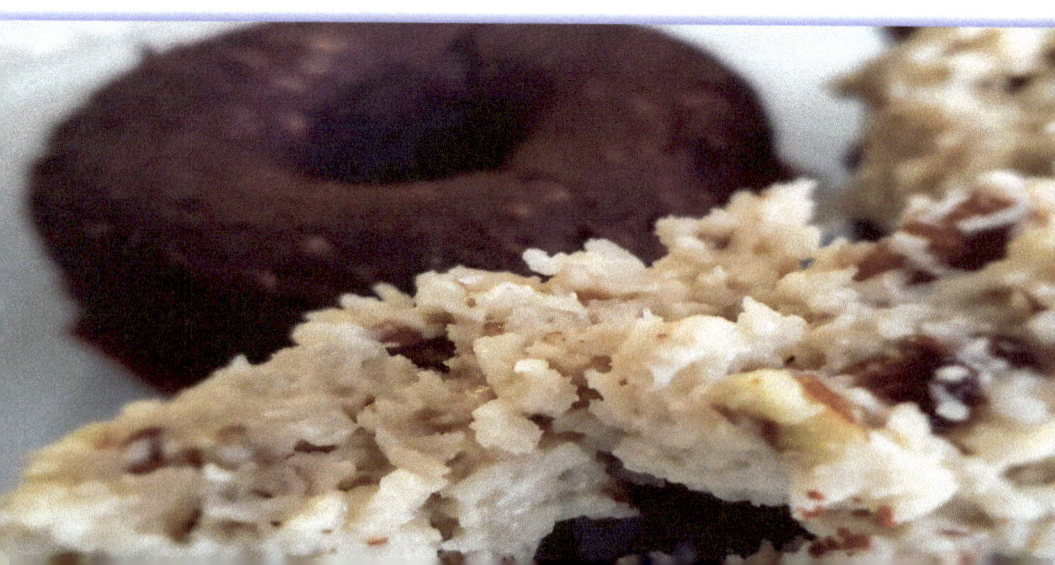

Celebration Cake

Preparation: *Soaking:* *Drying:* Makes 6-8
30 Min. *8-12 Hrs.* *8-12 Hrs.* Servings

Ingredients

Cake

- 5 c. pecans
- 3 c. dates, pitted
- 1 c. raw carob powder
- ½ tsp. Himalayan chrystal salt
- 1 c. buckwheat

Berry Syrup

- ½ c. favorite berries
- water if needed

Carob Icing

- 1 c. cashews
- ¾ c. water
- 1 inch vanilla bean or 1 tbsp. vanilla extract
- 5 tbsp. raw carob powder

Topping

- ¾ c. fresh berries in season

Directions

Soak pecans overnight, drain water off. Soak dates in enough water to cover for 30 minutes.

In a food processor, combine nuts and dates until smooth. Add carob, salt, and dry buckwheat that has been ground in a coffee grinder.

Divide cake mix into 3 equal parts. Form into rounds making sure they are about the same size and dry about 6 hours.

In a blender, mix berries and a little bit of water if needed, mix until syrup texture is reached. Pour into a bowl and set aside.

Using a blender, combine cashews, water, vanilla, and carob blend until fluffy.

Putting it together:

Place one round of cake batter on serving dish. Brush with some berry syrup. Spread carob icing on bottom layer.

Place 2nd round on top of icing and brush top with more of the syrup and spread more carob icing on top of the syrup. Place fresh berries on this layer, leaving enough for decorations on the top.

Place the 3rd round of cake on top of the berries and brush with remaining syrup. Use remaining icing to cover the cake. Decorate as desired using reserved berries and your imagination. Chill before serving.

Note

For winter omit the berries or use frozen.

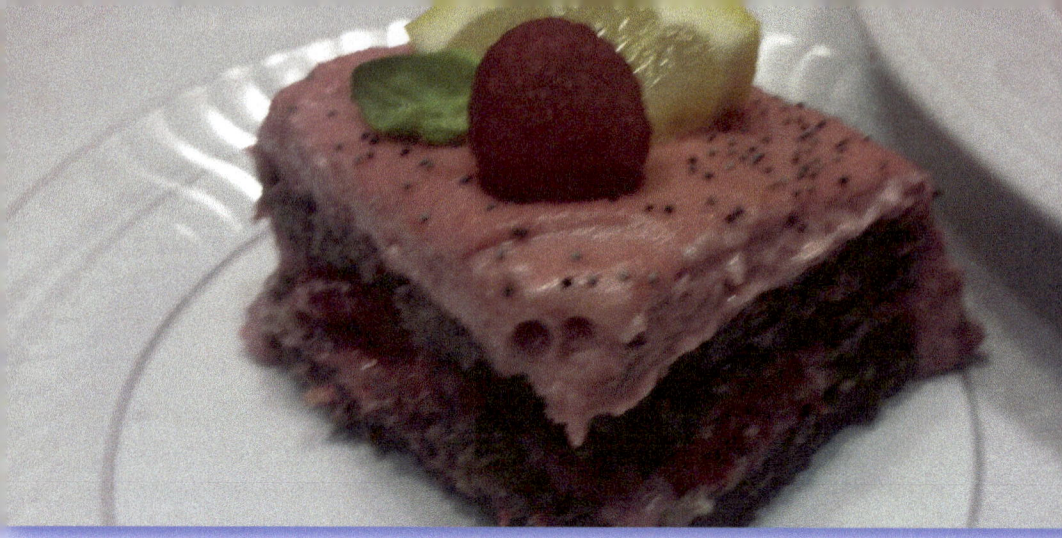

Raspberry Lemon Cake

Preparation: 20 Min. Drying: 2-6 Hrs. Makes 6-8 Servings

Ingredients

Cake

- 1 ½ c. cashews
- 1 ½ c. pecans
- ¼ c. raw liquid sweetener
- 2 lemons, juiced
- 1 inch vanilla bean or 1 tsp. vanilla extract
- ½ tsp. nutmeg
- 1 tbsp. poppy seeds

Raspberry Frosting

- 1 ½ c. macadamia nuts
- 1 lemon, juiced
- ¼ c. raw liquid sweetener
- 1 pint raspberries
- 1 inch vanilla bean or 1 tsp. vanilla Extract.

Topping

- ½ c. raspberries
- 2 tbsp. poppy seeds
- ½ lemon

Directions

In a food processor, combine macadamia nuts, pecans, raw sweetener, olive oil, lemon juice, vanilla, and nutmeg mix well. If cake is not firm enough, add up to 4 tbsp. slippery elm or coconut to thicken.

Form cake and set it aside. For a layered cake make sure rounds or squares are of equal size.

Place cake on nonstick dehydrator sheet and dry at 100°F. for about 3 hours flip it about half way through removing the nonstick dehydrator sheet.

In a blender, combine cashews, sunflower seeds, raw sweetener, lemon juice, raspberries, and vanilla. Blend until creamy and light.

Frost cake with raspberry frosting. Decorated with poppy seeds, whole raspberries and lemon wedges.

Pumpkin Cake

Preparation: 40Min. Drying: 4-6 Hrs. Makes 6-8 Servings

Ingredients

- 1 c. macadamia nuts
- 1 c. almonds
- ¾ c. raisins
- 1 c. pumpkin
- 1 tsp. Himalayan crystal salt
- 1 tsp. ground nutmeg
- 1 tsp. ground pumpkin pie spice
- 2 tsp. ground cinnamon
- 2 inches vanilla bean or 1 tbsp. vanilla extract

Directions

Soak almonds overnight. Peel brown skin off almonds while wet. May soak macadamia nuts 1-4 hours.

Combine macadamia nuts, walnuts, almonds, raisins, pumpkin, carrot, salt, nutmeg, cinnamon and vanilla in a food processor until evenly mixed.

Shape into rounds about ½ inch high, on a nonstick dehydrator sheet. Dehydrate for 4 hours. Flip and remove the plastic nonstick sheet and continue dehydrating at 100° F for about another 4 hours or until desired moisture is achieved.

Remove and decorate with Cream Frosting (page 110), pecans, and coconut.

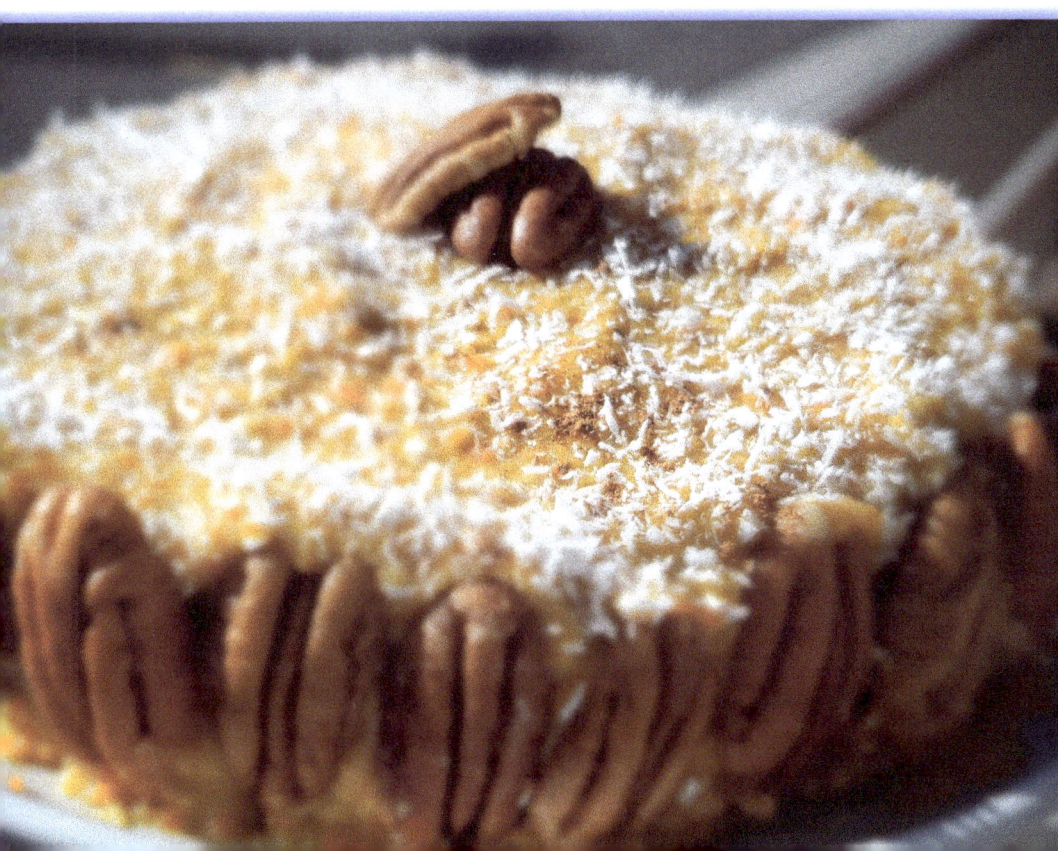

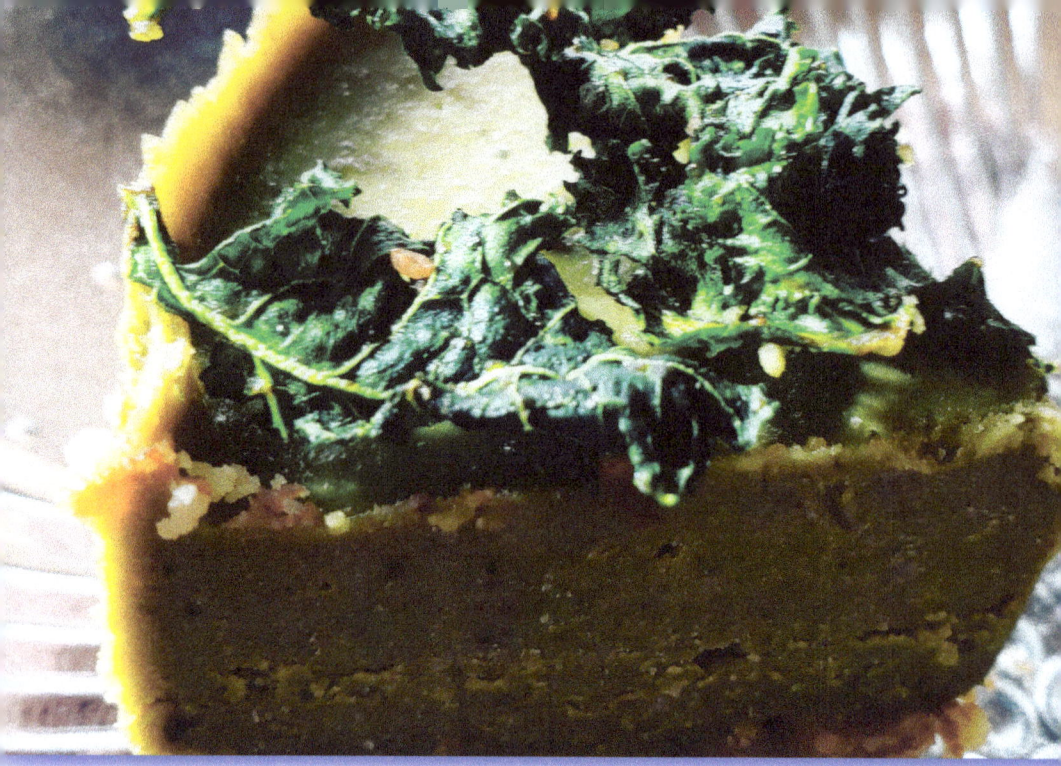

Sweet Kale Cheesecake

Preparation: 35 Min. Chill: 3-5 Hrs. Makes 6-8 Servings

Ingredients

Cheesecake

- ½ c. cashews
- ½ c. macadamia nuts
- 1 c. kale
- ½ c. zucchini
- ½ c. coconut oil
- ½ c. raw coconut nectar
- ¼ tsp. Himalayan crystal salt
- 2 tbsp. lemon juice
- ¼ c. water

Crust

- 1 c. pecans
- ½ c. dates

Note

Can be made with all cashews or macadamia nuts.

Directions

Place pecans, in a food processor add pitted dates and blend until well mixed. Press crust into a spring form pan.

In a food processor or high-power blender, place cashews, macadamia nuts, zucchini, kale, coconut oil, coconut nectar, lemon juice, and salt blend until smooth. Add water, as needed, to achieve a thick smooth texture.

Pour mixture onto crust and freeze for at least 5 hours. Decorate with candied kale (page 110). Keep refrigerated.

Pumpkin Cheesecake

Preparation: 30 Min.   *Chill: 1-3 Hrs.*   *Makes 6-8 Servings*

Ingredients

Crust

- ½ c. dates
- 1 c. pecans or walnuts

Filling

- 1 ½ c. cashews
- 2 c. pumpkin
- 1 lime, juiced
- ½ c. raw sweetener
- zest (peel) of lime
- 1 tbsp. pumpkin pie spice
- dash of Himalayan crystal salt
- ½ - 2 cups water as needed
- ½ inch vanilla bean or 1 tsp. vanilla extract

Topping

- ¼ c. cranberries
- ¼ c. raspberries
- 1 tsp. pumpkin pie spice
- 2 tsp. vanilla

Directions

In a food processor, combine dates and pecans or walnut until finely chopped. Press in pie plate or spring form pan and set aside.

In a blender combine cashews, shredded pumpkin, lime juice, sweetener (coconut nectar, agave, or honey), lime zest, pumpkin pie spice, vanilla, and salt blend until smooth. Adding water as needed to be thick and smooth.

Pour into crust and chill several hours before serving. Top with cranberry raspberry sauce.

In a food processor, pulse cranberries, raspberries, pumpkin pie spice, and vanilla until it is mixed. Should be chunky.

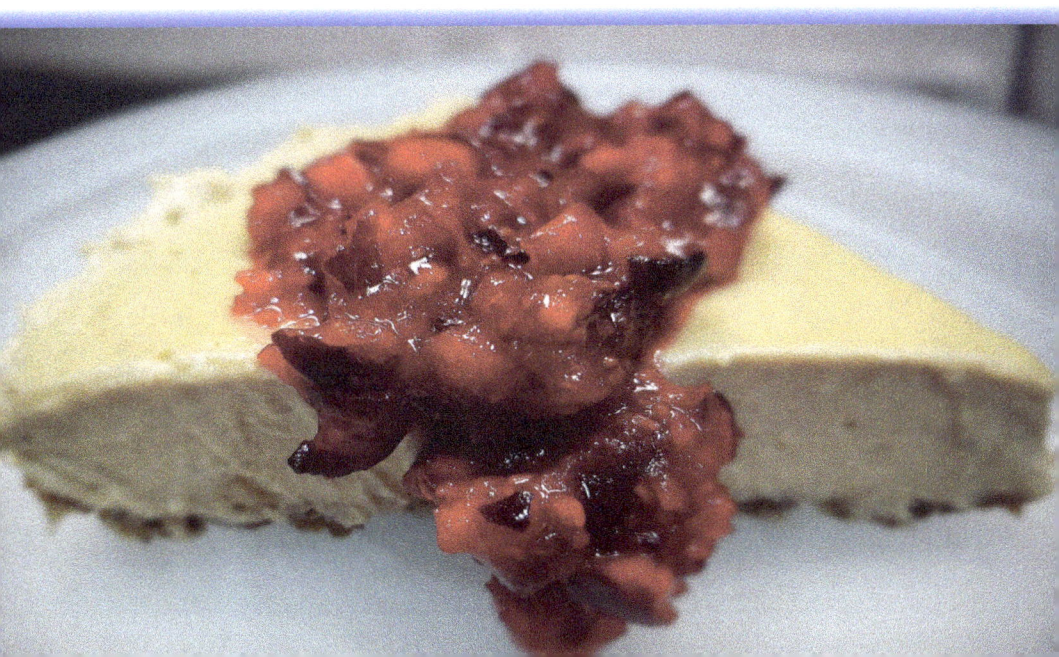

Mom's Apple Pie

Preparation: 20 Min.

Makes 4-6 Servings

Ingredients

Crust

- 1 ½ c. pecans
- ½ c. dates

Filling

- 6 c. apples
- ¼ lemon, juiced
- 1 tsp. nutmeg
- ½ tsp. cloves
- 1 inch vanilla bean or 1 tbsp. vanilla extract
- ¼ tsp. cold pressed olive oil
- ¼ tsp. turmeric
- ¼ tsp. Himalayan crystal salt
- ¼ c. raw coconut sugar
- ¼ c. raw almond butter

Crumb Topping

- 1 ½ c. macadamia nuts
- 1 ½ c. coconut, shredded

Directions

In a food processor, combine pecans and pitted dates combine until well mixed. Press into a plate and set aside.

Peel, core, and chop apple then place in a bowl. To apples add lemon juice, nutmeg, cloves, vanilla, turmeric, olive oil, coconut sugar, and almond butter gently mix and pour into pie plate.

In food processor, coarsely mix macadamia nuts, slowly add coconut until well mixed. Sprinkle over the top of the pie and let sit for an hour. Serve cold or dehydrate for about 4 hours if you wish at 100°F.

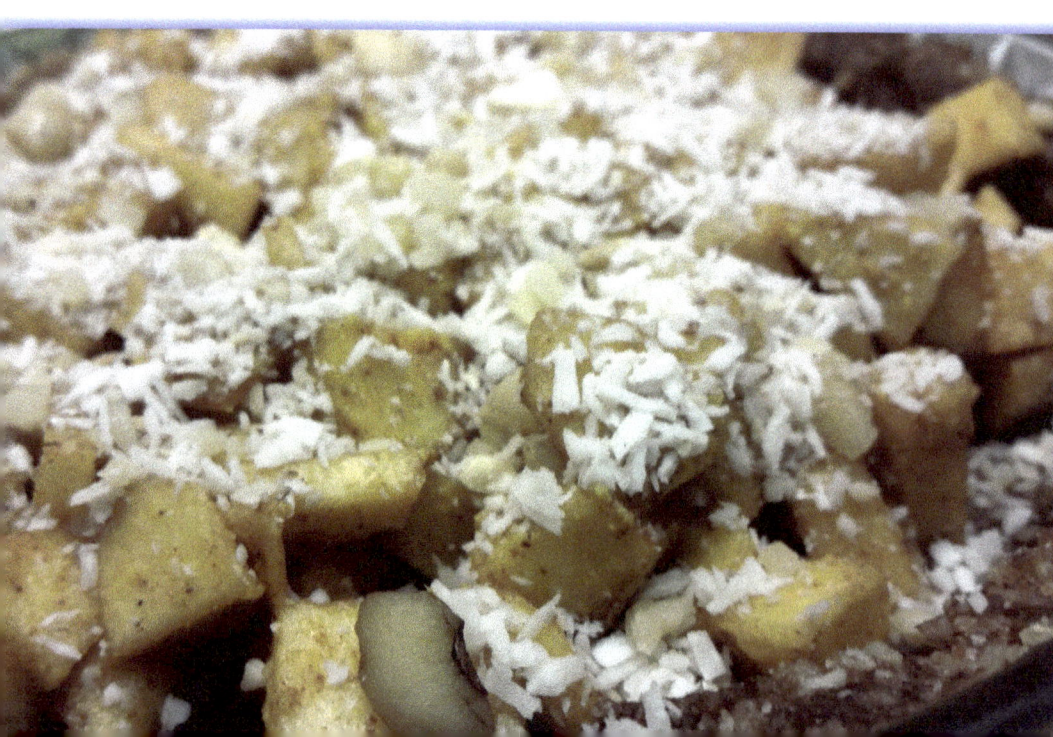

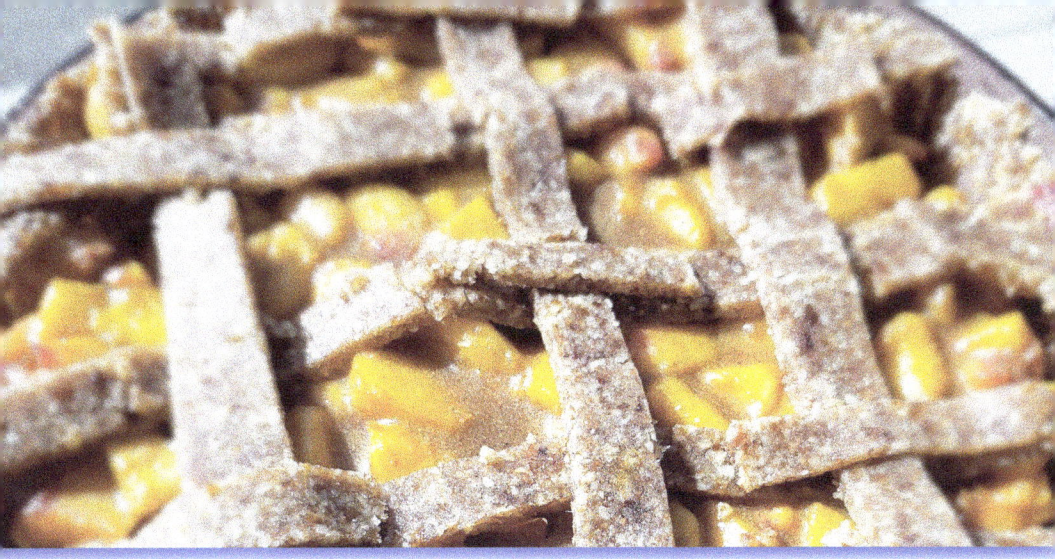

Peach Pie

Preparation: 20 Min. *Chill:* 1-4 Hrs. *Makes 4-6 Servings*

Ingredients

Crust

- 2 c. pecans
- 1 c. dates
- ¼ c. coconut flour

Filling:

- 5 c. peaches
- ¼ c. coconut oil
- ½ lemon, juiced
- 1 tsp. vanilla
- ½ c. raw coconut sugar
- ¼ tsp. cinnamon
- Pinch of nutmeg
- ¼ tsp. turmeric
- ½ tsp. Himalayan crystal salt
- 1 tbsp. phylum husk powder

Directions

Soak pecans overnight, drain water and place nuts, in a food processor along with pitted dates and coconut flour. Blend until well mixed. Press about ¾ of the crust into a pie plate set aside. Roll the remaining piecrust out into a square and cut strips to put on top of pie.

Peel and cut peaches and mix with lemon juice to prevent oxidation (turning brown).

Place coconut oil in a small jar with a lid. Place the jar, with lid on, in a bowl of warm water until coconut oil is liquid. Pour coconut oil in a bowl, stir in coconut sugar until it is well mixed add vanilla, cinnamon, nutmeg, turmeric, salt, and phylum husk. Pour mixture over peaches and gently mix.

Using a slotted spoon scoop out peaches from sugar mixture and place in the piecrust. There may be left over liquid in the bowl. May use leftover liquid in another recipe.

Palace cut piecrust strips over the top of the pie. Refrigerate pie for at least an hour before serving.

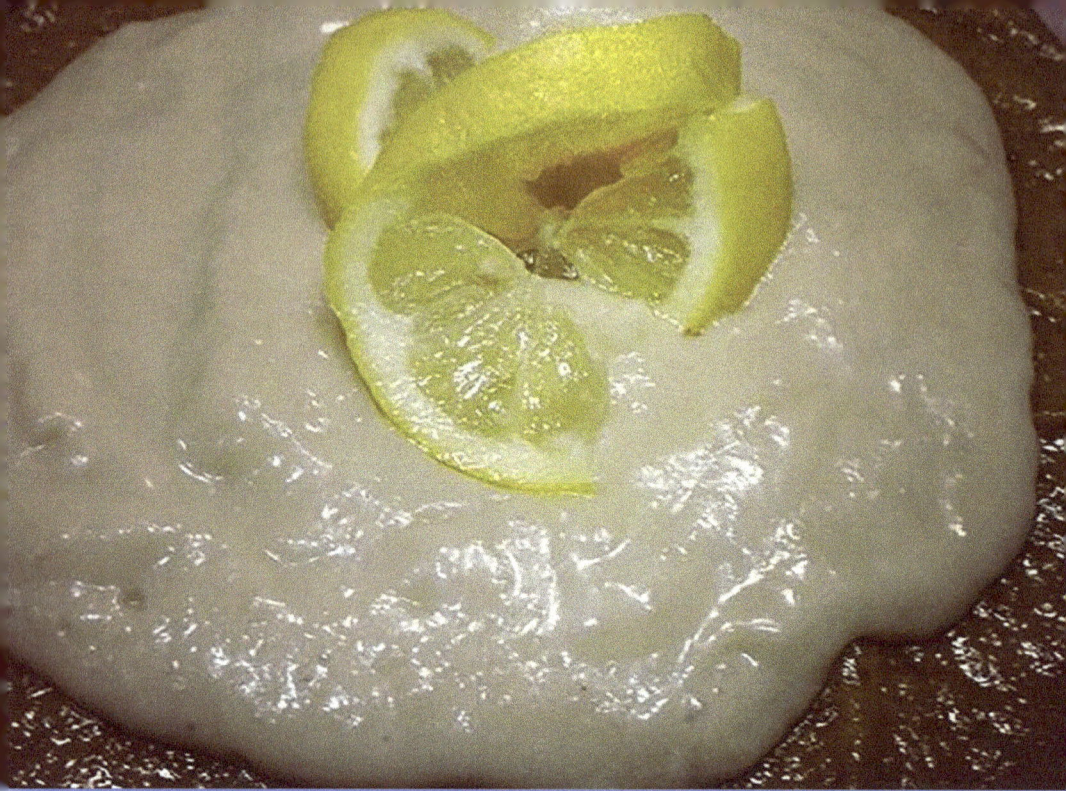

Lemon Pie

Preparation: 35 Min. Chill: 3-5 Hrs. Makes 6-8 Servings

Ingredients

Crust

1 ½ c. pecans
1 c. dates

Filling:

- 5 c. golden raisins
- 4. lemons, juiced
- 2 tbsp. lemon zest (peel)

Directions

Soak golden raisins in lemon juice and zest for 30 minutes.

Place soaked pecans in a food processor along with pitted dates mix until well blended. Press into a pie plate and set aside.

In a blender, combine raisins and lemon mixture until creamy smooth. Pour into pie plate and place into the refrigerator may top with coconut cream topping (page 142).

Fun Fact

Lemons were so popular during the gold rush that people were willing to pay $1.00 for one in 1849. About $30 today.

Blackberry Torte

Preparation: 20 Min. Chill: 1-3 Hrs. Makes 4-6 Servings

Ingredients

Crust
- ½ c. dates
- 1 c. pecans or walnuts

Filling
- 2 c. macadamia nuts
- 1 lime, juiced
- ½ c. raw liquid sweetener
- dash of Himalayan crystal salt
- ½ - 2 cups water as needed
- ½ inch vanilla bean or 1 tsp. vanilla extract

Topping
- 3 c. blackberries
- ¼ c. raw coconut nectar

Directions

Soak pecans overnight, drain off water and place nuts in a food processor with pitted dates. Mix until well combined then press into a pie plate or spring form pan and set aside.

In a blender, combine macadamia nuts, lime juice, coconut nectar, salt, and vanilla blend adding only the water needed to make the nuts creamy and smooth. Pour into pie plate and put in the refrigerator for 15 minutes.

In a blender, combine 1 cup blackberries, coconut nectar until creamy.

Remove torte from the refrigerator. Place remaining blackberries on the top of the pie. Gently pour the blackberry sauce over the top. Refrigerate for about an hour before serving.

Fun Fact

Some believe that the crown of thorns, placed on Christ's head at his crucifixion was made of blackberry brambles.

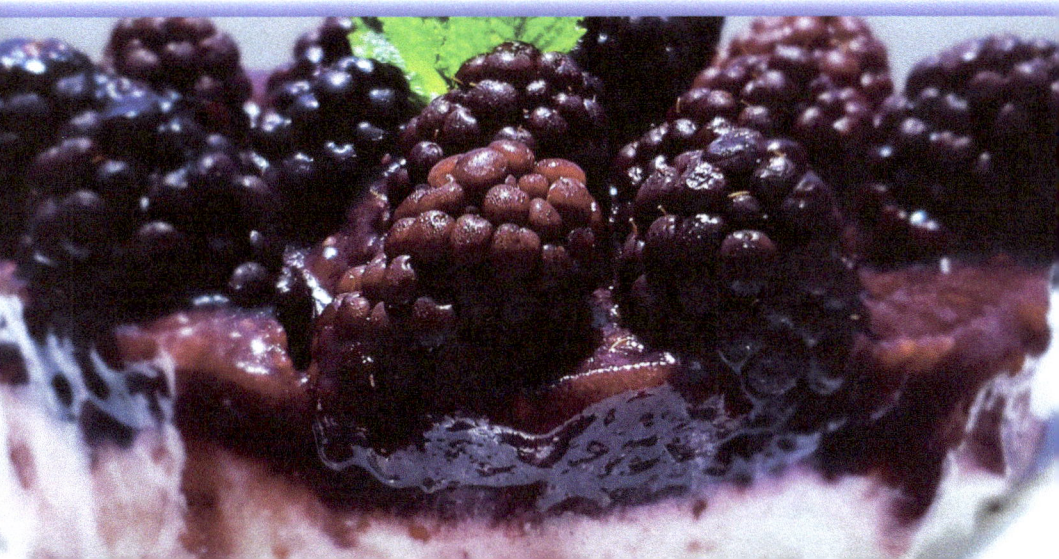

Candied Kale

Preparation: 20 Min.   *Drying:* 1-2 Hrs.   *Makes 4-6 Servings*

Ingredients

- 1 bunch kale
- 1 tbsp. cold pressed olive oil
- 3 tbsp. coconut nectar
- 1 tsp. Himalayan crystal salt

Directions

Remove kale leaves from stems and tear leaves into large pieces.

Wash and thoroughly dry kale pieces.

In a bowl, mix coconut nectar, olive oil and salt. Massage the oil mixture into kale.

Place kale on a dehydrator tray in a single layer and dry for about an hour. Chips should be crispy when done.

Coconut Sugar Bumps

Preparation: 20 Min.   *Drying:* 1-2 Hrs.   *Makes 4-6 Servings*

Ingredients

- 1 c. flaked oat groats
- ¾ c. raw coconut sugar
- 1 ½ c. raw almond butter

Note

Old fashioned rolled oats may be used instead, if no flaker is available.

Directions

In a bowl, combine flaked oats, almond butter, coconut sugar, and shredded coconut until well mixed.

Roll mixture into ½ inch balls and then roll in the coconut. Refrigerate for about a day to allow the flavors to mingle.

Cream Frosting

Preparation: 10 Min.   *Makes 6-8 Servings*

Ingredients

- 1 c. macadamia nuts
- ½ c. raw coconut oil
- ½ c. raw liquid sweetener
- ¼ - ¾ c. water

Directions

In a blender, combine macadamia nuts, coconut oil, raw liquid sweetener, until smooth adding only enough water until desired thickness and smoothness is achieved.

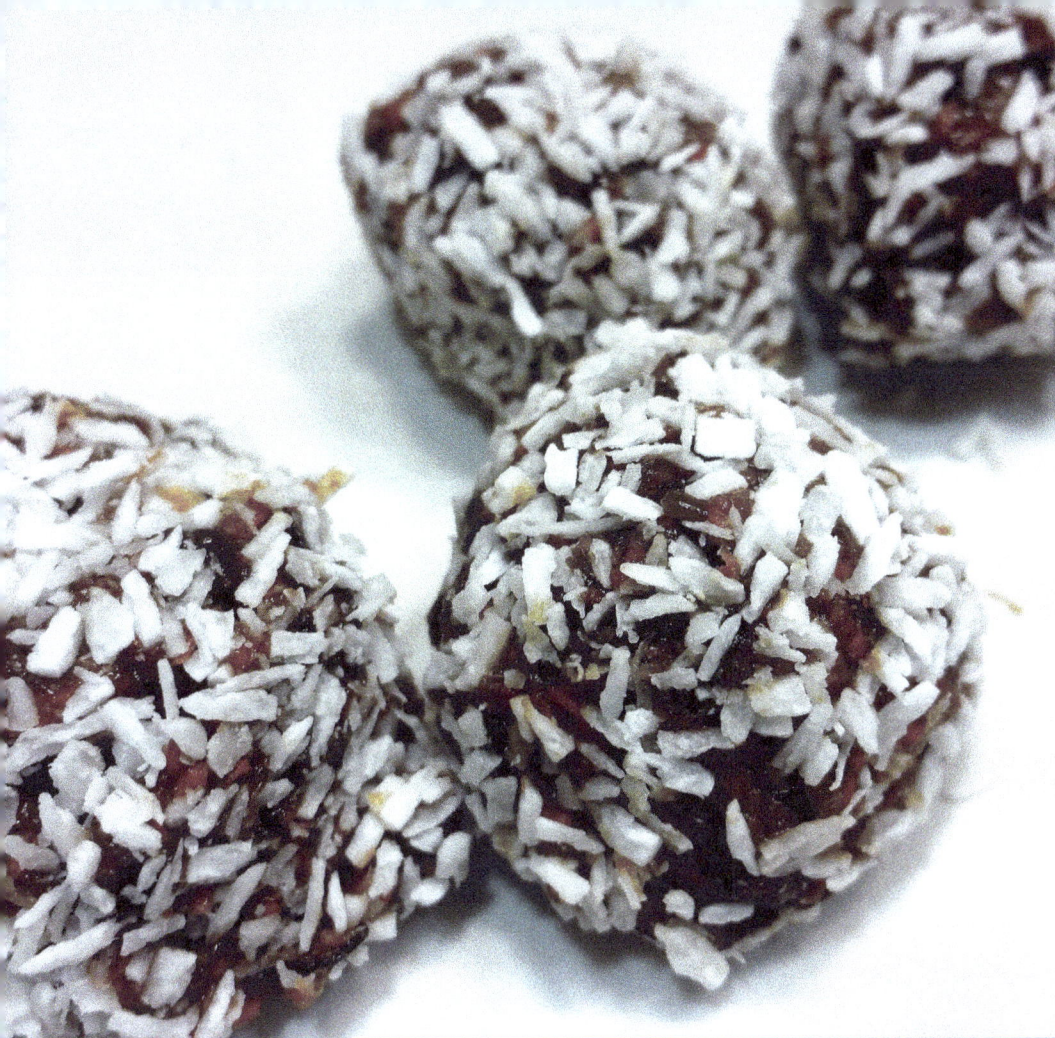

Flax Balls

Preparation: 15 Min.   Chill: 2-4 Hrs.   Makes 4-6 Servings

Ingredients

- 1 c. prunes, pitted
- 1 c. raisins
- 1 c. carrots, grated
- 1 tbsp. flax seed
- ¼ c. cold water
- ¼ c. coconut, grated

Directions

In a food processor, combine prunes, raisins, carrots, and flaxseed ground in a coffee grinderuntil well mixed.

Wet hands in cold water and form balls about 2 tablespoons in size. Roll balls in coconut and place on a cookie sheet. Refrigerate for 2 to 4 hours before eating. Keep all extras in the refrigerator and enjoy.

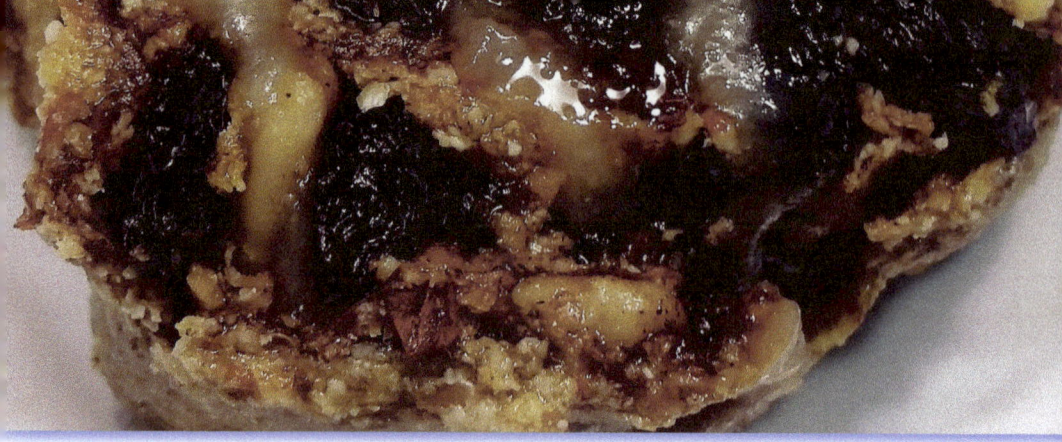

Cinnamon Rolls

Preparation: 20 Min. Soaking: 8-12 Hrs. Drying: 4-6 Hrs. Makes 4-6 Servings

Ingredients

Bread
- 4 c. almond pulp
- 1-2 c. golden flax,
- 1 c. dates, pitted

Filling
- 1 c. walnuts or pecans
- ¼ c. cinnamon, ground
- 2 c. raisins
- ½ c. raw coconut sugar
- 4 tbsp. cold press olive oil
- ½ tsp. turmeric
- 1 tsp. Himalayan crystal salt
- ½ inch vanilla bean or ½ tbsp. vanilla extract

Directions

Soak pecans and walnuts overnight then drain off water. Soak dates in water for 20 minutes, save date water for later use

In a food processor, combine almond pulp left from making almond milk, golden flax seeds ground in a coffee grinder, and dates combine until well mixed. Adding date water as needed. Rollout a rectangle on some parchment paper or a non-stick dehydrator sheet and set aside.

In a food processor, coarsely chop walnuts, pecans, and cashews.

In a small container, mix olive oil, turmeric, vanilla, and salt. Brush on bread then sprinkle with cinnamon and coconut sugar top off with raisins and nuts.

Roll bread tightly and cut into slices. Place on a dehydrator sheet at 105°F for about 5 Hours. Drizzle cream frosting over the top.

Fun Fact

In Ancient Egypt, cinnamon was a highly prized and was valued more than gold. It was used in food, drink and as an embalming agent.

Black Bottom Coconut Bars

Preparation: 20 Min. Chill: 1-3 Hrs. Makes 6-8 Servings

Ingredients

Black Bottom

- 1 c. unrefined coconut oil
- ¾ c. raw coconut nectar
- 1 c. raw carob powder
- 1 inch vanilla bean or 2 tbsp. pure vanilla
- 2 c. walnuts or pecans

Coconut Topping

- 2 c. macadamia nuts
- ¾ c. coconuts oil
- 1 tsp. turmeric
- 2 c. coconut, shredded
- 1 inch vanilla bean or 2 tsp. pure vanilla extract

Fun Fact

Coconuts are not a nut but actually a stone fruit, like peaches.

Directions

Melt coconut oil in a bowl over a warm pan of hot water or double broiler keeping the temperature of the oil about 100°F.

To coconut oil, add coconut nectar, carob powder, and vanilla. Stir until it starts to get thick. Add chopped nuts to carob mix. Press into bottom of a large cake pan cover it and set it aside.

In a food processor, mix macadamia nuts, coconut oil, turmeric, shredded coconut, and vanilla. Mix until very well combined and almost creamy.

Spread coconut mixture over the top of carob black bottom mixture; place in the refrigerator until hard. Cut into bars and enjoy.

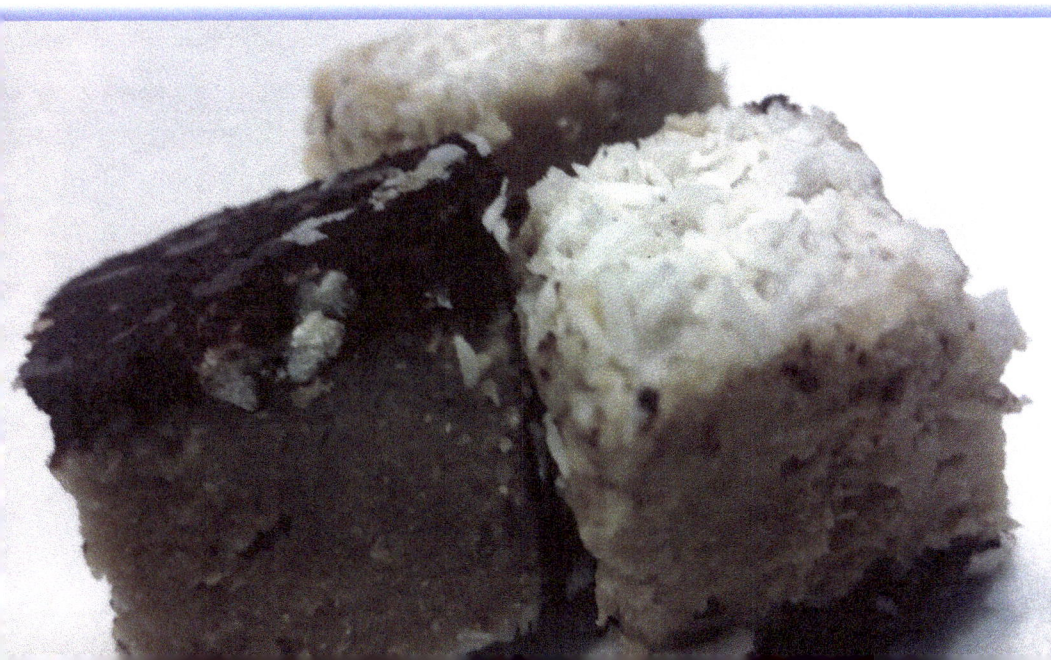

Fudge Sickle

Preparation: 15 Min.   *Chill:* 2-4 Hrs.   *Makes 4-6 Servings*

Ingredients

- 2 c. sesame seed milk (page 142)
- 2-4 bananas, frozen
- ¼ c. raw liquid sweetener
- 4 tbsp. raw carob powder

Fun Fact

11-year-old boy accidently invented popsicles when he left a sweet drink on the porch overnight which froze. That summer he sold his frozen treat for 5 cents a peace.

Directions

Peel then freeze bananas. Make the sesame seed milk.

In a blender, place sesame seed milk, frozen bananas, raw sweetener, and carob powder blend until thick and smooth. Pour into paper cups, with a popsicle stick in the center, freeze.

Enjoyed eating by peeling off the paper cup and holding it by the stick.

Blond Ambition

Preparation: 20 Min.   *Chill:* 1-4 Hrs.   *Makes 4-6 Servings*

Ingredients

- 1 ½ c. sesame seeds, don't soak
- ¾ c. coconut, shredded
- ½ c. raw tahini
- ¼ c. raw almond butter
- ½ - ¾ c. raw liquid sweetener

Fun Fact

I have had several of my blonde friends ask, "Why Blond Ambition?" Then they taste it and say "Blond Ambition's a good name."

Directions

Combine tahini, almond butter, and sweetener in a bowl. Slowly add sesame seeds and coconut, mix well.

Spread mixture into a pan, smoothing with a spatula, or use a small scoop and make balls.

Pace mixture in the refrigerator until firm, about 2 hours. If in a pan, cut into triangles or bars and enjoy.

Peanut Butter Bars

Preparation: 40 Min.

Soaking: 8-12 Hrs.

Drying: 10-14 Hrs.

Makes 6-8 Servings

Ingredients

Bars

- 2 c. walnuts
- 2 c. oat groats
- ½ c. raw tahini
- ½ c. raw almond butter
- 3 tbsp. cold pressed olive oil
- 1 tsp. Himalayan crystal salt
- 1 tsp. turmeric
- ¾ c. raw liquid sweetener
- 1 inch vanilla bean or 1 tbsp. pure vanilla

Peanut Butter

- ½ c. raw tahini
- ½ c. raw almond butter
- ¼ c. raw liquid sweetener

Carob Frosting

- 3 tbsp. raw liquid sweetener
- ¾ c. raw carob powder
- 2 tsp. pure water

Directions

Make sure to use dry nuts, if they are not, the texture will be wrong.

Grind oat grouts in a coffee grinder and place in food processor. Place walnuts, ½ cup tahini, ½ cup almond butter, olive oil, salt, turmeric, and sweetener in the food processor and mix until it looks like cookie dough. Dehydrate at 100 F for about 8 hours and place in the refrigerator for 5 hours.

In a bowl, mix ½ cup tahini, ½ cup almond butter, and sweetener mix with a spoon until smooth. Spread onto bars.

Place carob in a small bowl, add sweetener and mix slowly with a spoon adding water as needed to achieve a creamy frosting. Spread on top of the peanut butter.

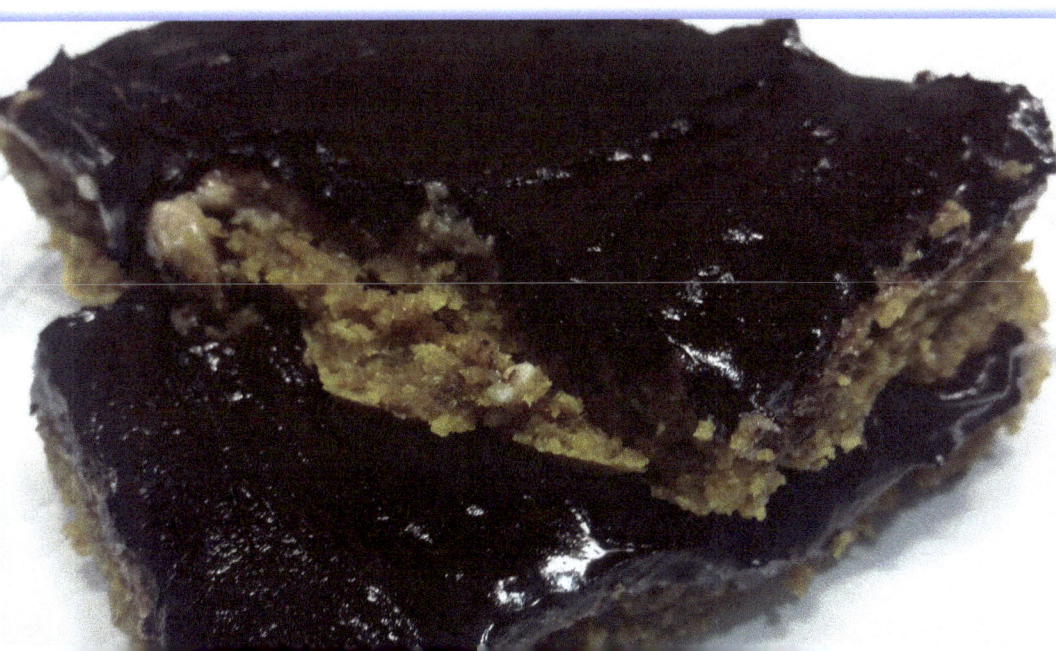

Carrot Brownies

Preparation: 40 Min. Soaking: 8-12 Hrs. Drying: 8-12 Hrs. Makes 6-8 Servings

Ingredients

- 1 ½ c. carrots
- 3 c. walnuts
- 2 c. cashews
- 2 c. dates
- ½ tsp. Himalayan crystal salt
- 2 tsp. cinnamon
- 1 c. raw carob powder
- ¼ c. coconut oil
- ½ inch vanilla bean or 1 tsp. vanilla extract

Directions

Soak walnuts overnight drain water off and place nuts in food processor with shredded carrots, cashews, and dates combine until well mixed. Incorporate salt, cinnamon, carob, oil, and vanilla to the food possessor mix.

Scoop out contents of food processor and shape it into a square until it is about an inch thick. Place on non-stick dehydrator sheet on a tray.

Dehydrate about 4 hours then flip, pull off non-stick sheet, and continue drying another 4 hours.

Serve with Carob Frosting (page 99) for a white topping, use Cream Frosting (page 110).

Variation

For mint brownies add spirulina and mint to cream frosting. Spread over the brownie then top with carob frosting.

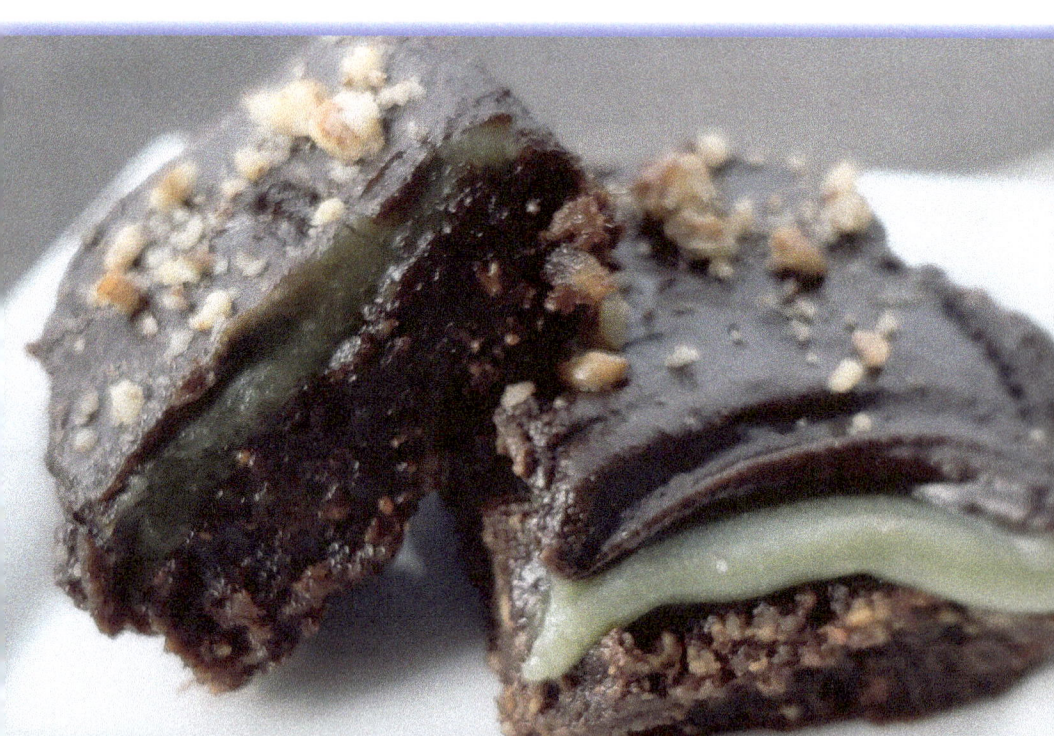

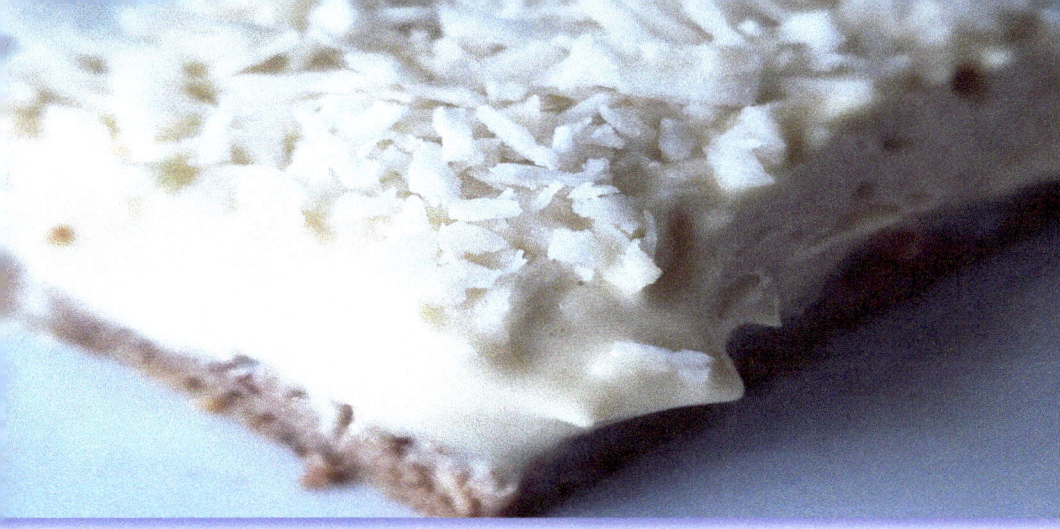

Lemon Bars

Preparation: 20 Min. *Drying:* 4-6 Hrs. *Chill:* 8-12 Hrs. *Makes 6-8 Servings*

Ingredients

Crust

- ¾ c. pecan
- ¾ c. walnuts
- ¼ c. dates
- 1 tbsp. vanilla

Filling

- 2 c. cashews
- 1 young coconut meat
- ¼ c. Irish moss gel
- ½ c. coconut water
- 3 lemons, juiced
- 2 lemons, zest
- ½ c. coconut nectar
- ¼ tsp. turmeric powder
- ½ c. shredded coconut

Directions

Soak dates in water for about 20 minutes, drain water off dates, save water for later use.

In a food processor, combine pecans, walnuts, dates and vanilla.

Shape crust about ½ inch think. Can be done be done using hands or in a spring form pan. Place in dehydrator and dry for 4-6 hours.

In a blender, combine lemon juice, Irish moss gel, lemon zest, coconut nectar, coconut meat, cashews, and turmeric until creamy.

Place lemon mixture over the crust. Sprinkle shredded coconut over the top and place in refrigerator overnight.

Fun Fact

During the Pacific War of 1941-45, coconut water was used to give emergency plasma transfusions to wounded soldiers.

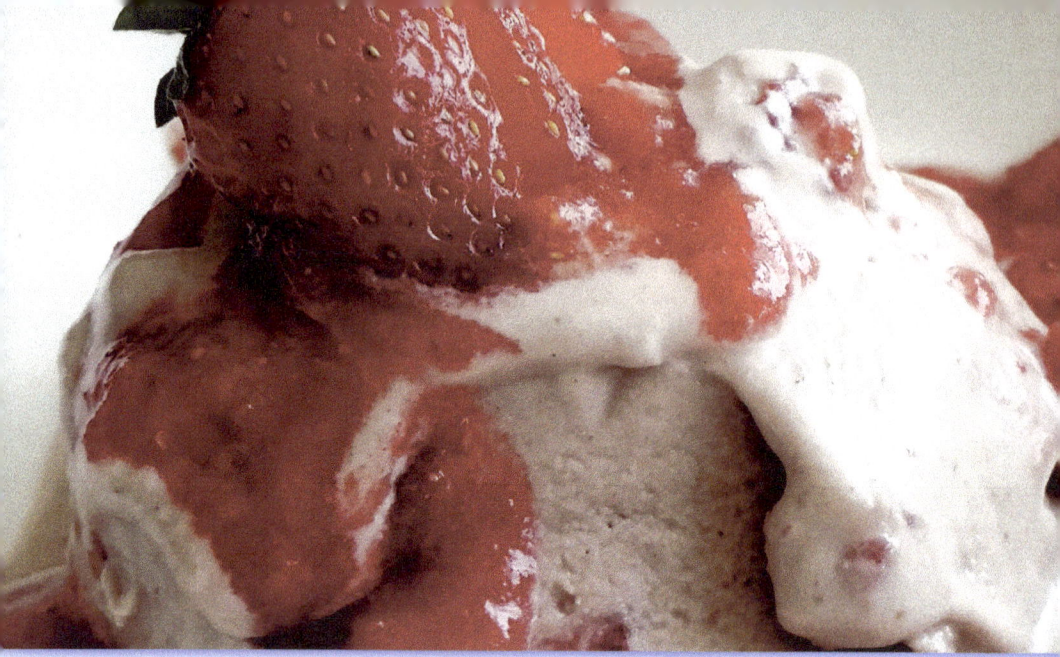

Strawberry Ice Cream

Preparation: 15 Min. Chill: 20-30 Min. Churning: 20-30 Min. Makes 6-8 Servings

Ingredients

- 1 c. cashews
- ½ c. raisins
- 1 ½ c. water
- ¼ c. coconut nectar
- 1 tsp. raw vanilla powder or 1 tbsp. vanilla extract
- 1 tbsp. coconut oil
- 1 c. strawberries

Directions

Soak raisins for 20 minutes. Save water to use latter.

Place ½ cup strawberries and raisins, coconut nectar, vanilla, coconut oil, and cashews into a blender and combine until smooth. Use raisin water if needed.

Using a cheesecloth over a container to strain out large particles for a very smooth base.

Place mixture into freezer for 10-15 minutes. If you skip this step, it will not set up property in the ice cream maker. The mixture should be cool but not to the point where ice crystals begin to from.

Stir in reaming strawberries. Pour mixture into ice cream maker it should reach ideal consistency about 20 minutes.

Note

Use a traditional ice cream maker to churn mixture or freeze mixture in ice cube trays then blend them in a food processor.

Chocolate Ice Cream

Preparation: 15 Min. Chill: 20-30 Min. Churning: 20-30 Min. Makes 6-8 Servings

Ingredients

- ½ c. cashews
- ½ c. macadamia nuts
- ¾ c. dates, pitted
- 2 ½ c. water
- 1 tsp. raw vanilla powder or 1 tbsp. vanilla Extract
- 1 tbsp. coconut oil
- 3 tbsp. carob powder

Note

Do not use ice cream maker bowl to freeze or chill the mixture. The base will freeze to the bowl and ruin the ice cream.

Use a traditional ice cream maker to churn mixture. If you wish you can freeze the mixture in ice cube trays then bend them in a food processor.

Fun Fact

Vanilla is the only fruit-bearing member of the orchid family.

Directions

Pit and soak dates for 20 minutes. Save the water to use later.

Place cashews, macadamia nuts, dates, vanilla, coconut oil, and carob into a blender and combine until smooth. Add date water as needed to achieve smoothness. If more water is need then use pure water.

Using a cheesecloth strain out all large particles for a very smooth base. Place mixture into the freezer for 10-15 minutes. If you skip this step, it will not set up property in the ice cream maker.

The mixture should be cool but not to the point where ice crystals begin to from. Pour mixture into the ice cream maker and churn.

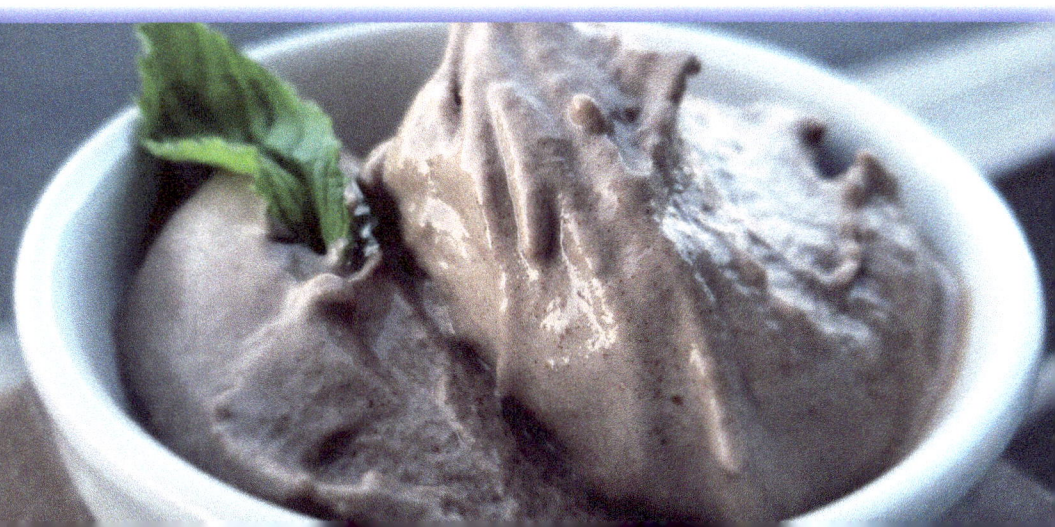

Chocolate Dipped Ice Cream Sandwich

Preparation: 20 Min. Chill: 8-12 Hrs. Makes 6-8 Servings

Ingredients

- chocolate or other flavor vegan ice cream

Sandwich

- ¾ c. raw almonds (or other nuts of choice)
- 5 soft Medjool dates
- 3 tbsp. raw carob powder
- ½ tbsp. vanilla powder
- pinch of salt

Carob Dipping Sauce

- 4 tbsp. cacao butter
- 5 tbsp. coconut oil
- ½ - 1 c. raw carob powder
- 1 tbsp. vanilla powder
- pinch Himalayan crystal salt

Notes

Carob powder is available at most health food and whole food grocery stores. Store it in airtight, opaque containers. Choose glossy, dark brown pods, without cracks and pits when buying whole fresh carob pods.

Fun Fact

The Bible says that John the Baptist's ate locust and wild honey during his time in the wilderness. Middle Eastern tradition calls carob tree pods St. John's Bread because he ate locust bean pods (carob pod) not the insect.

Directions

Make vegan ice cream.

Combine almonds, carob powder, and salt in food processor until a fine powder is created. Add dates and vanilla. Process until a uniform, sticky dough is formed add water if needed to help cookie dough stick together.

Roll out dough about ¼ inch thick. With a cookie cutter cut out an even number of cookies. Place the dough in the freezer to set for 20 minutes.

Remove chocolate cookies from freezer, and place a large spoonful of ice cream on half of the cookies. Use the other half to create sandwiches, press cookies together to even out ice cream middles. Place back in the freezer until solid and can be handled, about 20 minutes.

Make chocolate dip by melting the cacao butter and coconut in a bowl placed over very hot water, add vanilla and salt then mix. Slowly add carob stirring to keep lumps from forming. Continue adding carob until it is a thick enough for dipping.

Dip ice cream stuffed cookies half-way then freeze until solid. Store sandwiches in a sealed container in freezer.

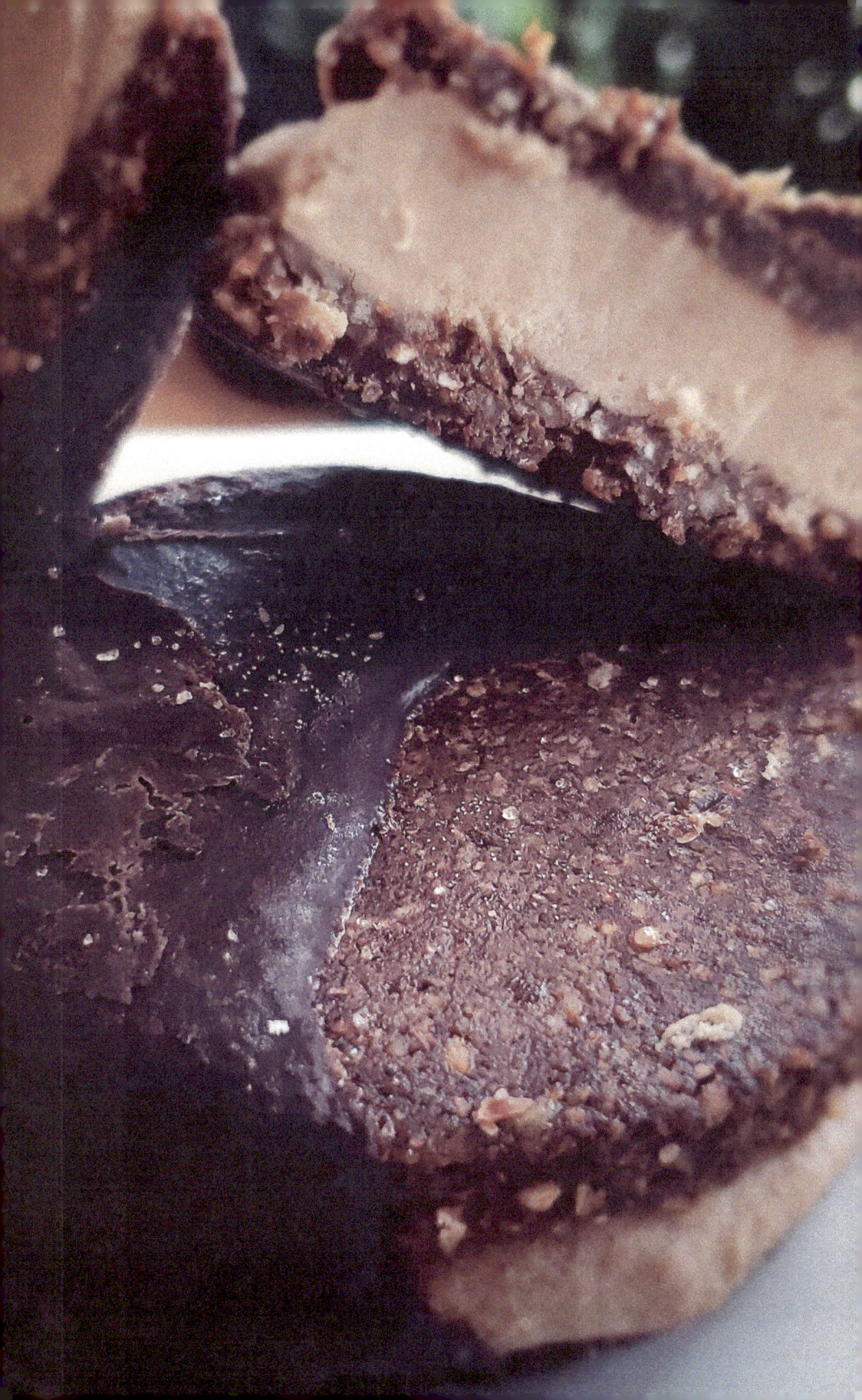

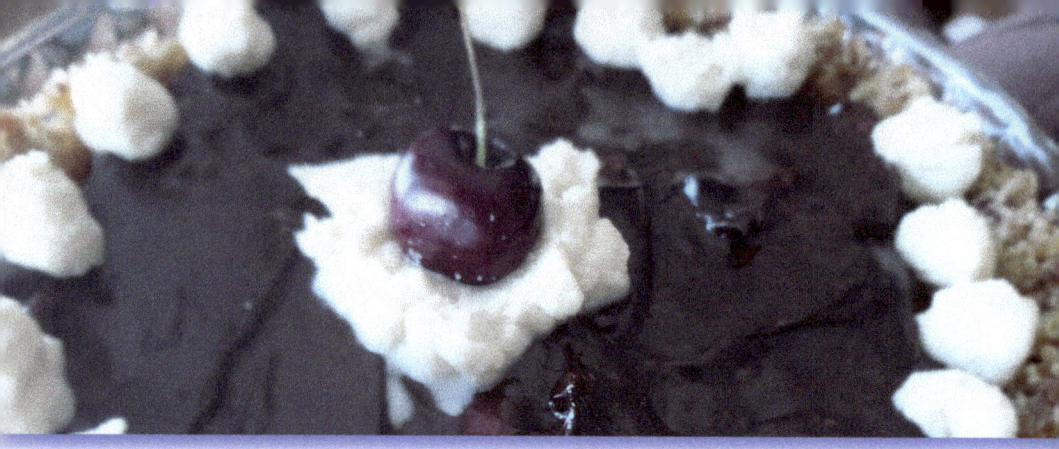

Chocolate Cherry Pie

Preparation: 20 Min.

Makes 4-6 Servings

Ingredients

Crust
- 1 ½ c. pecans
- ½ c. dates

Filling
- ¾ c. fresh cherries

Chocolate Pudding
- 3 ripe avocadoes
- ¾ c. raw liquid sweetener
- 1 c. raw carob powder
- ½ inch vanilla bean or 1 tsp. vanilla extract

Topping
- 1 c. cashews
- water as needed

Directions

Place pecans in a food processor along with pitted dates; blend until well mixed and press into a pie plate. Set aside.

In a blender, place avocadoes that have been peeled and pitted, raw coconut nectar, and vanilla. Blend until creamy smooth adding a little bit of water as needed for it to be creamy. You want it to be thick like pudding.

Slice and pit cherries reserve a few for garnish. With a spoon stir remaining cherries in chocolate pudding. Pour pudding on crust. Place in refrigerator for at least an hour.

In a blender, combine cashews, sweetener, and water until it is light and fluffy. Pour the topping over the filling and place a couple of cherries on the top of the pie.

Variations

1) For a chocolate pie, omit cherries.

2) For a chocolate banana pie, in place of cherries use sliced bananas on the bottom of the crust and then add the pudding filling.

Strawberry Pie

Preparation: 20 Min. Drying: 3-4 Hrs. Chill: 3-4 Hrs. Makes 4-6 Servings

Ingredients

Crust

- ½ c. dates, pitted
- 1 ½ c. macadamia nuts
- ¼ tsp. Himalayan crystal salt
- 1 c. coconut, shredded

Filling

- 6 c. strawberries

Glaze

- 3 tbsp. agar agar flakes
- ½ c. strawberries, juiced
- ½ c. hot water
- ¼ c. cold water
- ½ c. raw liquid sweetener

Directions

In a food processor, combine dates, macadamia nuts, salt and coconut until crumbly and well mixed. Press into pie plate; dehydrate crust for 4 hours.

Place whole or sliced strawberries in crust.

Stir agar agar into cold water and allow to set 1 minute. Bring hot water to a boil and simmer for 2 minutes, add to the cold water mix and let cool.

In a separate bowl, stir together strawberry juice and sweetener; pour cooled agar agar liquid over the juice mixture stir. Pour over strawberries in pie plate and refrigerate for 3 hours.

May top with whipped coconut cream (page 142) if desired.

Fun Fact

Ancient Romans used strawberries to treat depression, fever, and sore throats.

Note

Agar-agar is produced from red algae seaweed that is 100% natural. It is completely odorless and tasteless. It is used as a stabilizing and thickening agent.

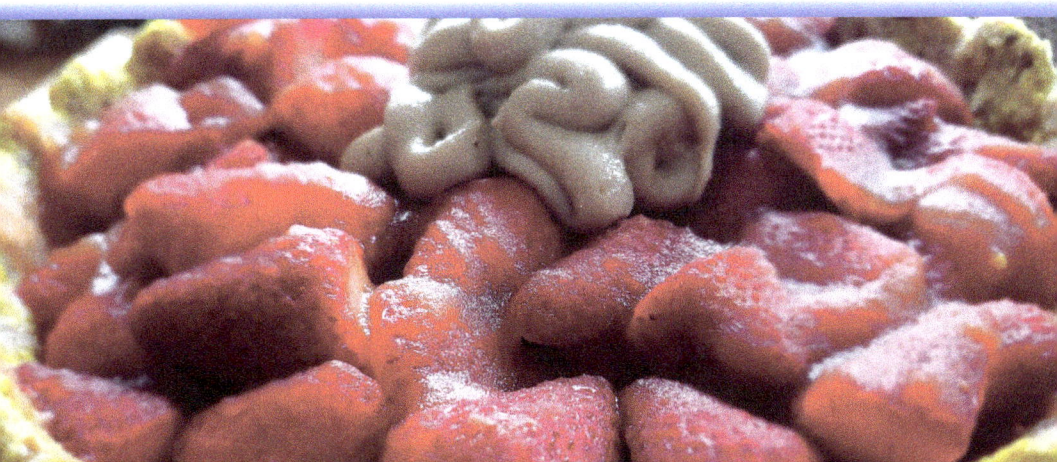

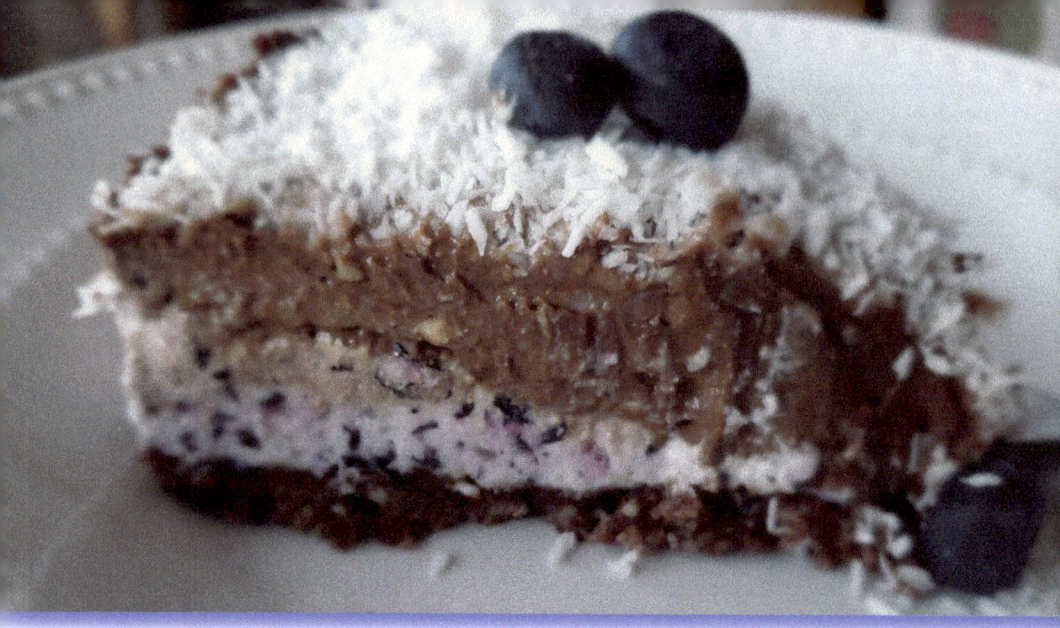

Mississippi Mud Pie

Preparation: 30 Min.   *Chill:* 3-5 Hrs.   *Makes 6-8 Servings*

Ingredients

Crust
- ½ c. dates, pitted
- 1 ½ c. macadamia nuts
- ¼ tsp. Himalayan crystal salt
- ½ c. coconut, shredded
- 1 tbsp. raw carob powder

Filling
- 3 ripe avocados
- ¾ c. liquid raw sweetener
- 1 c. raw carob powder
- ½ inch vanilla bean
- ½ c. coconut oil

Topping
- ¼ c. coconut, shredded
- whipped cashew cream
- 2 tbsp. cacao bar (optional)
- vegan fruit cream cheese with blueberries

Note
For winter omit berries or use fruit in season

Directions

Make vegan fruit cream cheese with blueberries (page 148).

In a food processor, combine dates, macadamia nuts, salt, carob and coconut until crumbly and well mixed. Press into a pie plate.

Spread the vegan fruit cream cheese over the bottom of the pie crust.

In a food processor, combine peeled and pitted avocados, sweetener, carob, vanilla, and coconut oil until smooth. Pour into pie pan and refrigerate for 30 minutes.

Top with cashew cream (page 143) and shredded coconut may shred carob bar over the top.

Pumpkin Candy

Preparation: 15 Min.
Freezing: 4-8 Hrs.
Makes 6-8 Servings

Ingredients

Candy

- 1 small sugar pumpkin
- ¾ c. raw tahini (sesame butter)
- ¼ c. pure water
- ½ inch vanilla bean or 1 tbsp. vanilla extract
- 1 lemon, juiced
- 1 tbsp. pumpkin pie spice
- 2 tsp. cinnamon
- 4 tbsp. raw liquid sweetener

Carob sauce

- 1 c. coconut oil
- 1-2 c. raw carob powder
- ½ c. raw liquid sweetener
- water if needed

Directions

Peel, seed, and shred pumpkin. Place shredded pumpkin in food processor and blend until smooth. Add, vanilla, lemon juice, pumpkin pie spice, cinnamon, and sweetener to pumpkin mix well.

In a small bowl, mix coconut oil, carob, and sweetener and mix, slowly add water, until desired thickness is achieved.

Scoop pumpkin mix into party cups cover with Carob Sauce. Place in freezer and serve frozen.

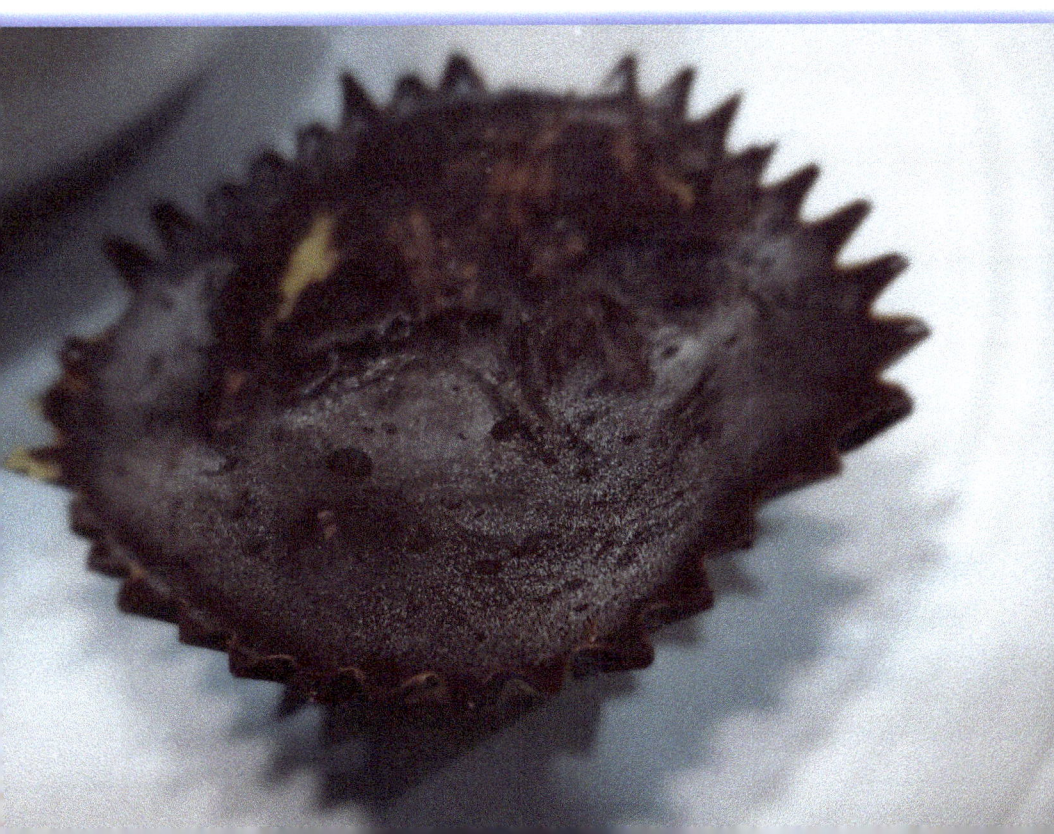

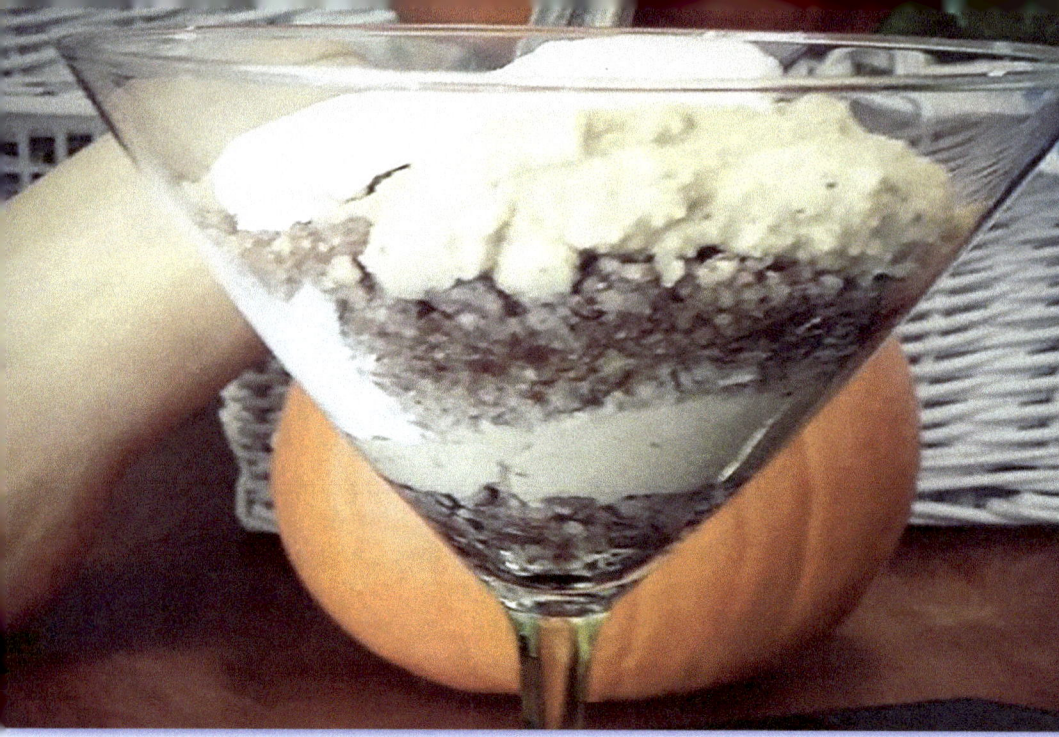

Pumpkin Parfait

Preparation: 20 Min. *Soaking:* 8-12 Hrs. *Makes 4-6 Servings*

Ingredients

- 2 c. pecan nuts, soaked
- 1 c. dates
- 1 small sugar pumpkin
- ¾ c. raw tahini (sesame butter)
- ¾ c. water
- ½ inch vanilla bean (may use 1 tbsp. vanilla extract if desired)
- 1 lemon, juiced
- 1 tbsp. pumpkin pie spice
- 2 tsp. ground cinnamon
- 1 c. cashew cream (page 142)

Directions

Make cashew cream and set aside.

Soak pecans overnight. Drain off water and place pecans and dates into food processor and mix until finely mixed. Set aside.

Peel, seed and shred pumpkin. Place pumpkin in blender and mix until smooth, add tahini, vanilla, lemon juice, pumpkin pie spice, and cinnamon mix well.

Spoon a layer of pumpkin mixture into bottom of a champagne or wine glass. Top with a layer of nuts and dates, and finally a layer of whipped cream. Repeat process until glass is full ending with the whipped cream.

Fun Fact

The word parfait is French origin meaning something perfect.

Carrot Ginger Cookies

Preparation: 10 Min. *Drying:* 3-5 Hrs. *Makes 6-8 Servings*

Ingredients

- 1 c. carrots
- 2 c. walnuts/pecans
- 1 ½ c. dates
- ½ c. raisins
- 3 tbsp. ginger, ground
- 3 tsp. cinnamon, ground
- 3 tsp. all spice
- 8 tbsp. coconut sweetener
- raw coconut flour as needed

Directions

Soak nuts overnight. Drain off water and place nuts in a food processor.

Add pitted dates and raisins to nuts along with ginger, cinnamon, and all spice. Combine until well mixed.

If dough is not sweet enough add coconut sweetener. If it is too wet, add coconut flour to get to cookie dough texture.

Drop round of the dough on nonstick dehydrator sheet and then flatten with a fork. Place cookies in dehydrator and dry for about 3 hours or until the desired dryness is achieved. Flip cookies half way through the drying and remove the nonstick sheet.

Fun Fact

Ground ginger root has a higher nutritional value than raw ginger root.

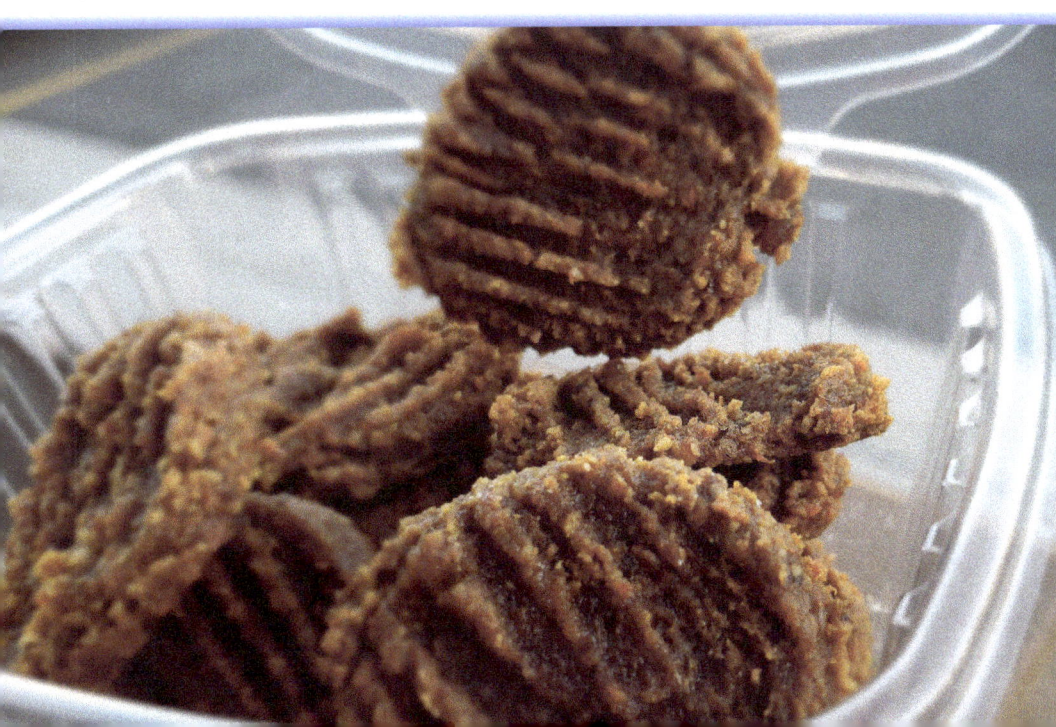

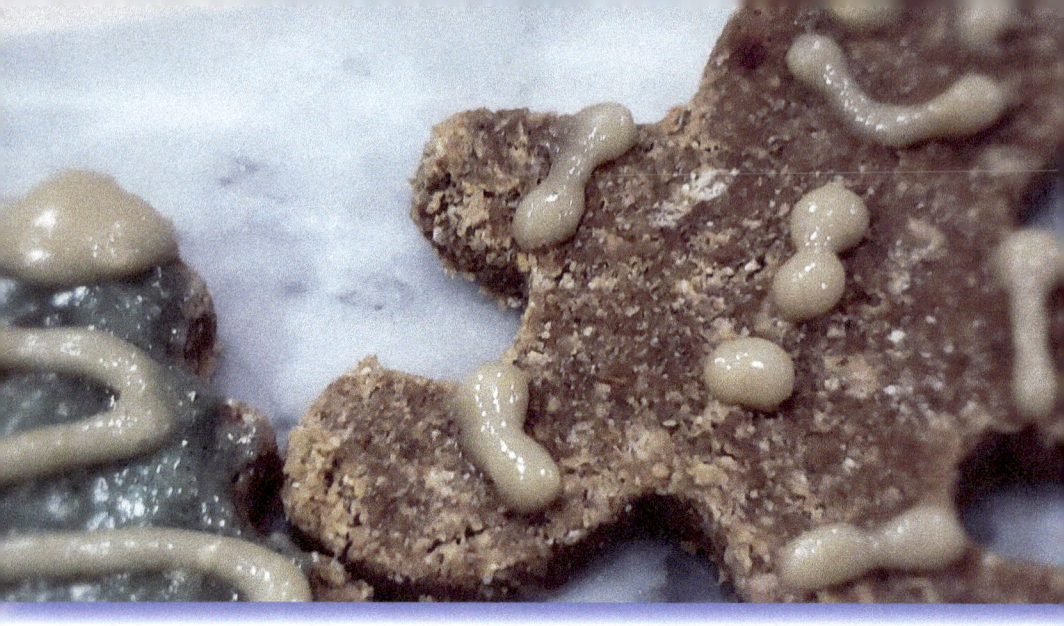

Soft Gingerbread Cookies

Preparation: 30 Min. Drying: 4-8 Hrs. Makes 6-8 Servings

Ingredients

- 1 c. dates
- 1 c. buckwheat
- ½ c. flax seed
- ½ tsp. allspice
- 1 tsp. cinnamon, ground
- ¾ tsp. cardamom, ground
- ¼ tsp. Himalayan crystal salt
- ½ tsp. clove, ground
- ½ c. coconut nectar
- 1 tbsp. ginger
- ½ c. raw coconut flour
- cashew cream frosting (page 143, optional)

Directions

Soak buckwheat overnight. Drain off water. Place dates in a food processor and mix, add soaked buckwheat continue mixing until well combined.

Grind flax seed in a coffee grinder then add to food processor with the buckwheat. Add allspice, cinnamon, cardamom, salt, clove, ginger, and coconut nectar mix until well combined.

Incorporate coconut flour, or buckwheat flour made from dried ground buckwheat, sprinkle some coconut flour on counter. Place dough from food processor on counter and knead adding more coconut flour as needed until the dough is firm and looks like cookie dough.

Roll dough out to about ¼ inch thick and using a cookie cutter, cut cookies. Place on nonstick dehydrator sheet and dry for about 2 hours. Flip and remove the nonstick sheet and continue drying for another 2-4 hours until the desired texture is achieved. After dry make cream frosting and decorate the cookies.

Fudge

Preparation: 15 Min. *Chill: 2-4 Hrs..* *Makes 6-8 Servings*

Ingredients

- 1 c. unrefined raw coconut oil
- ¾ c. raw cocoa butter
- 1 c. raw liquid sweetener
- 1 c. raw carob powder
- 1 inch vanilla bean or 2 tbsp. pure vanilla
- ½ c. walnuts or pecans
- pinch cayenne
- pinch salt

Directions

Melt coconut oil and cocoa butter in a warm pan or a double boiler over hot water; make sure internal temperature of the coconut oil does not go above 100°F.

To melted coconut oil, and cocoa butter add coconut nectar or raw liquid sweetener, carob, and vanilla and mix until everything is very smooth, and it starts to get thick mix in chopped pecans.

Spread fudge in cake pan cover and refrigerate for at least an hour. Cut it into pieces keep any leftovers in the refrigerator.

Banana Date Kebabs

Preparation: 10 Min. *Makes 6-8 Servings*

Ingredients

Kebabs

- 8 large pitted dates
- 2 tbsp. raw pistachios, chopped
- 1 tbsp. raw carob powder
- 1 tsp. coconut oil
- ½ orange, juiced
- 2 large bananas

Sweet Kebab Dipping Sauce

- 1 young coconut
- 2 tsp. vanilla or ¼ inch vanilla bean
- coconut water
- 1 tsp. coconut oil
- 1 tsp. raw coconut nectar

Directions

Combine coarsely chopped pistachios with carob powder, coconut oil, and 2 tablespoons orange juice. Stuff each date with pistachio mixture.

Cut bananas into 6 slices and roll in orange juice. Place 3 banana chunks and 2 dates making sure the dates are oblong on a skewer.

Dipping sauce

In a blender, combine young coconut meat, vanilla, coconut oil, and coconut nectar adding only enough coconut water for the mixture to become creamy.

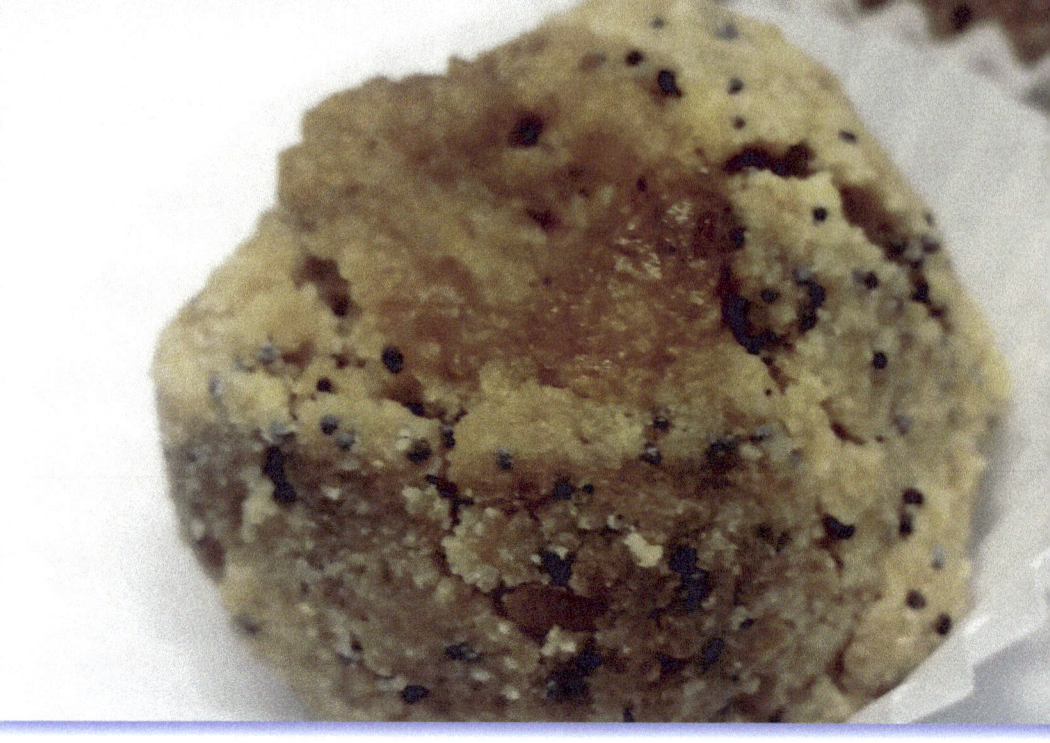

Lemon Poppy Muffins

Preparation: 20 Min. *Soaking:* 8-12 Hrs. *Drying:* 6-8 Hrs. *Makes 6-8 Servings*

Ingredients

- 1 c. cashews
- 1 c. almond pulp, left over from making milk
- 1 lemon, juiced
- 1 c. dates
- 1 tbsp. lemon zest (peel)
- 1 tbsp. poppy seeds
- 1 tsp. Himalayan crystal salt

> **Fun Fact**
>
> Leaves of a lemon tree can be used to make tea.

Directions

Using a food processor, mix cashews, almond pulp, lemon, salt, poppy seeds, lemon zest, and dates until well mixed then place in a bowl.

Drop dough onto a nonstick dehydrator sheet using a spoon or scoop. Place into dehydrator at 105°F for about 4 to 6 hours.

Flip muffins and carefully remove nonstick dehydrator sheet. Continue drying another 4 to 6 hours until desired moisture is obtained.

Note

Remember that the larger the muffins are the longer they will take to dry and the higher risk of them fermenting before they dry.

Apple Carrot Muffins

Preparation: 20 Min. *Soaking:* 8-12 Hrs. *Drying:* 6-8 Hrs. *Makes 6-8 Servings*

Ingredients

- 1 c. buckwheat
- 1 c. almond pulp, from making milk
- 1 c. carrot pulp, left over from juicing
- ¾ c. dates
- 1 c. raisins
- ½ c. apples, chopped
- ½ c. walnuts, soaked and dried chopped
- 1 tbsp. cinnamon
- 1 tsp. cardamom
- 1 tsp. cloves

Directions

Soak buckwheat and walnut overnight in separate bowls. Drain water off walnuts and buckwheat.

Using a food processor, mix buckwheat, almond pulp, walnuts, and dates until well mixed.

Move buckwheat mixture to a bowl, add raisins, apples, cinnamon, cardamom, and cloves, mix wilth a spoon until everything is well combined.

Drop dough onto a nonstick dehydrator sheet using a spoon or scoop. Place into dehydrator at 105°F for about 4 to 6 hours.

Flip or turn muffins over and carefully remove the nonstick dehydrator sheet. Continue drying another 4 to 6 hours until the desired moisture is obtained.

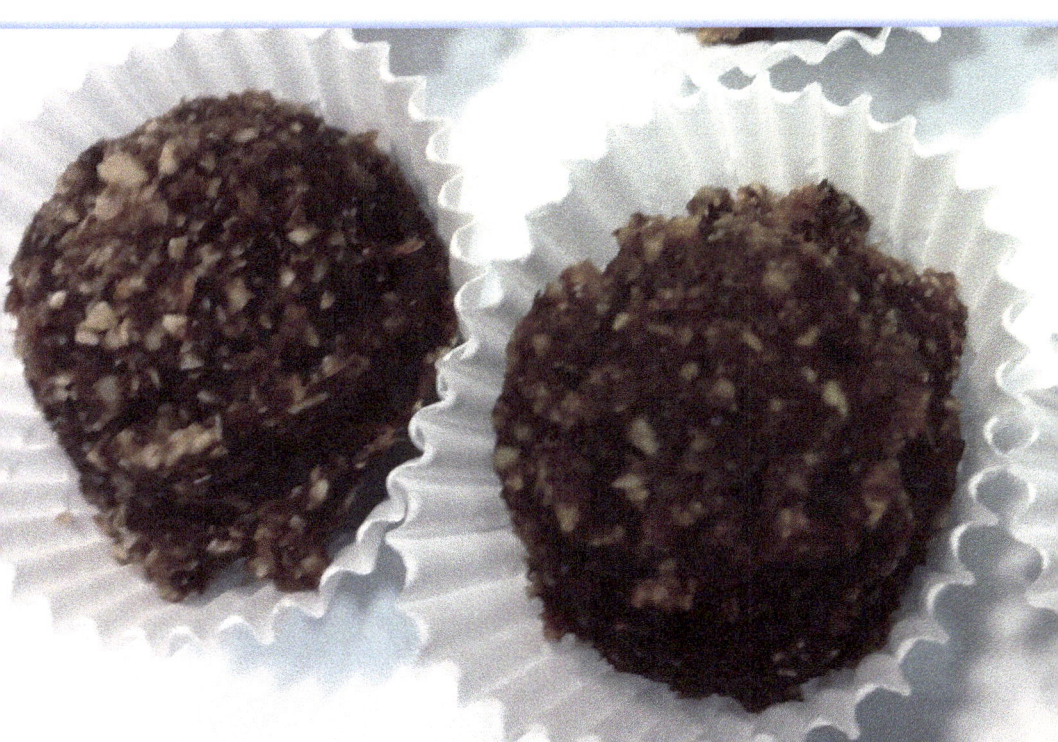

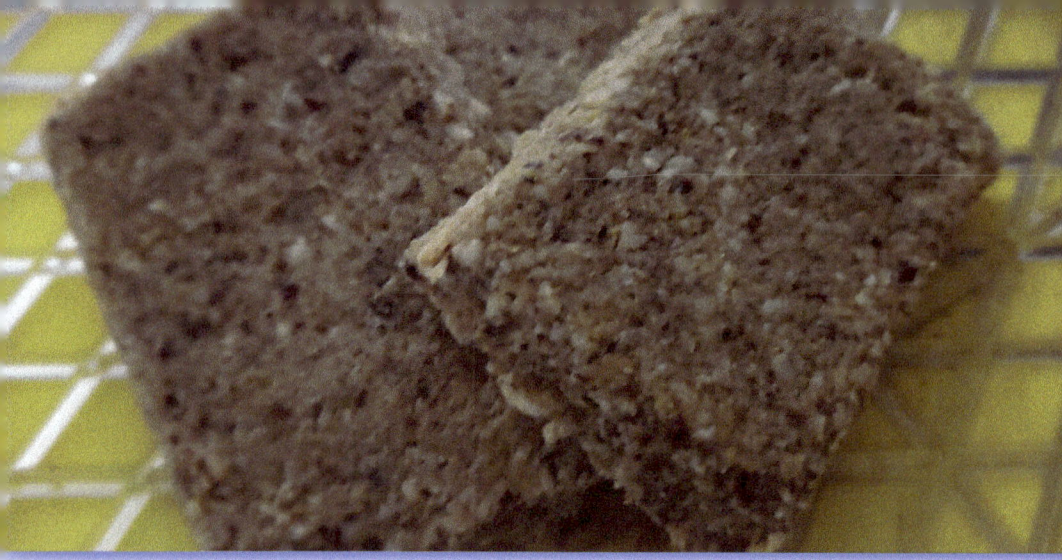

Corn Bread

Preparation: 20 Min. Soaking: 8-12 Hrs. Drying: 4-8 Hrs. Makes 6-8 Servings

Ingredients

- 2 c. almonds
- ½ c. cashews
- 1 c. hazelnuts
- 1 c. golden flax seed,
- 2 c. corn kernels, fresh or frozen
- ¼ c. raw liquid sweetener
- 2 tsp. Himalayan crystal salt
- 1-2 cloves garlic
- pure water as needed

Directions

In two separate bowls, soak almonds and hazelnuts overnight. Drain water off nuts. Place almonds and cashews into a food processor and blend adding water as needed until it looks like a dough. Place in a bowl and set aside.

In a food processor, place corn kernels, hazelnuts, garlic, salt, and raw sweetener. Combine until well mixed adding water as needed to achieve semi creamy state. Place in the same bowl with the almond and cashew mixture and gently mix.

Grind golden flaxseed in a coffee grinder. Slowly add flax meal to bowl ingredients and combine very well. Let sit for 5 to 10 min.

Spread mixture to about a ¼ of an inch thick and place on a dehydrator tray with nonstick dehydrator sheet. Score, or lightly cut into rectangles pieces.

Dry at 105°F for about 3 hours. Turn over and carefully remove nonstick dehydrator sheet. Continue drying for approximately 3 more hours. The bread is done when it still moist and easy to lift.

Rye Bread

Preparation:	Soaking:	Drying:	Makes 6-8
30 Min.	8-12 Hrs.	12-24 Hrs.	Servings

Ingredients

- 1 c. brown flax seeds
- ½ c. buckwheat
- ½ c. rye
- 1 medium onion
- 1 c. celery
- 2 tbsp. coriander
- ½ c. pure water
- ¼ c. cold pressed olive oil
- 1 tbsp. turmeric
- 1 tbsp. Himalayan crystal salt
- ½ c. raisins
- ½ lime, juiced

Directions

Soak buckwheat and rye overnight, drain off water and place into a food processor. Grind dry flax in a coffee grinder and set aside.

To food processor add onion, celery, raisins, lime juice, olive oil, until well mixed. Slowly add ground flax.

On non-stick dehydrator tray spread dough out until it is about a half an inch thick. Using a bread slice cookie cutter or score (lightly cut) bread with a knife, place bread onto a dehydrator sheet.

Dehydrate at 100° F for about 24 hours, flip bread about halfway.

Fun Fact

Unlike other grains, rye grows in poorer soil and colder climates. Traditionally, rye bread has a stronger taste and is chewier than wheat bread.

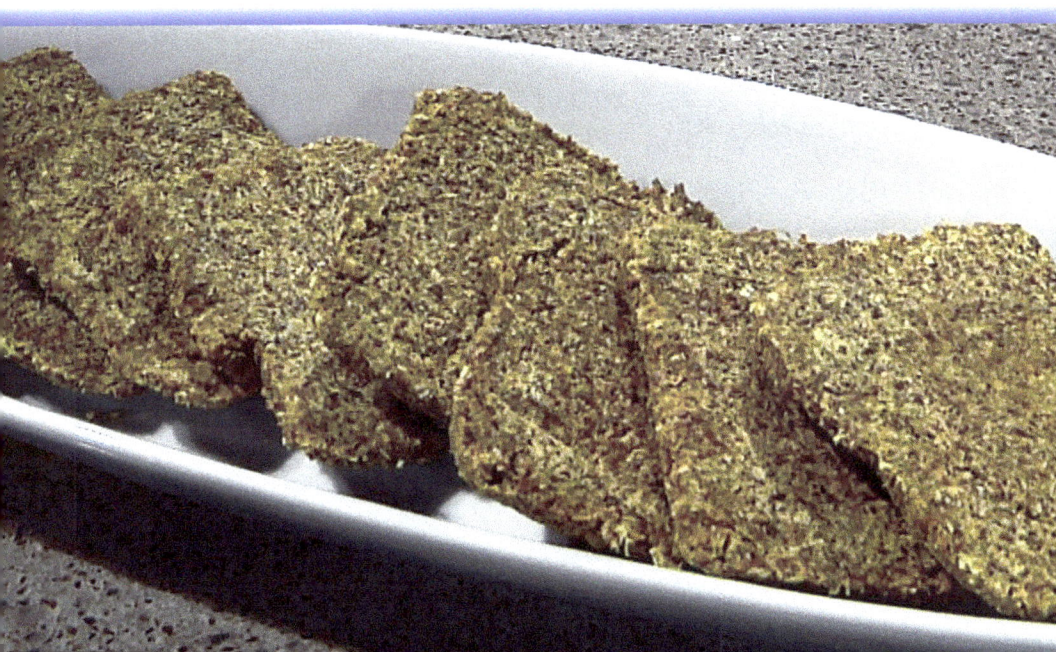

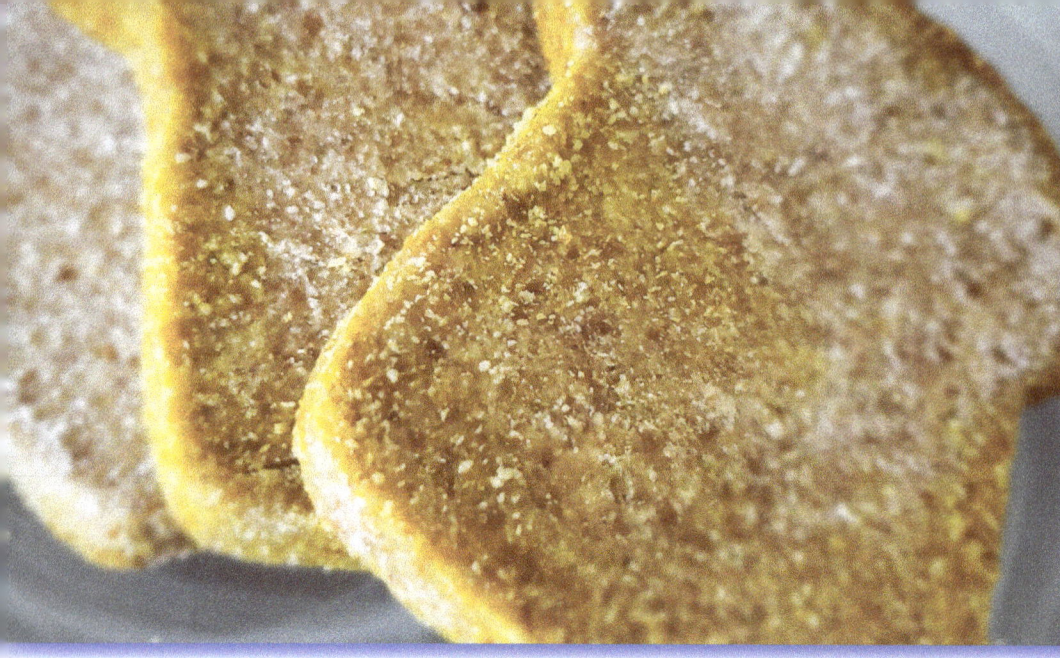

Nancy's Bread

Preparation: 20 Min.　　Soaking: 8-12 Hrs.　　Drying: 8-12 Hrs.　　Makes 6-8 Servings

Ingredients

- 1 c. gold flax
- 1 c. buckwheat, sprouted
- 1 tsp. Himalayan crystal salt
- 1 c. coconut flour

Directions

Soak buckwheat overnight, drain off water. In a food processor, combine buckwheat, ground flax, and salt. Mix until a thick dough, like a bread dough, is made.

Use coconut flour or ground buckwheat flour or to thicken dough if it is too sticky in the food processor.

Knead dough on counter or thin cutting board, use coconut flour to keep it from sticking to the counter or your hands.

Roll dough about a ¼ of an inch thick. Use a bread cookie cutter or cut into rectangles pieces and place on a dehydrator tray using a spatula. Dry for about 1 hour and 100°F.

Fun Fact

Flax is a native plant of the Mediterranean and has been used as a food item for well over 5,000 years with documented use in Babylon. It ranges in color from deep amber to golden yellow.

Hazelnut Bagels

Preparation: 30 Min.   *Drying:* 8-12 Hrs.   *Makes 6-8 Servings*

Ingredients

- 1 c. buckwheat
- ½ c. raw coconut four
- ½ c. flaxseeds
- 1 c. hazelnuts
- 2 tbsp. chia seeds
- ¾ c. zucchini, peeled
- 2 tbsp. coconut nectar
- 1 lemon, juiced
- 1 c. water
- ¼ c. cashews
- 2 tbsp. nutritional yeast (optional)

Directions

Place dried hazelnuts in a food processor and mix until a flour is formed. Grind flaxseeds and buckwheat in a coffee grinder and add to the food processor, along with chia seeds and set aside.

In a blender, place zucchini, coconut nectar, lemon juice, water, cashews, and nutritional yeast mix until creamy.

Pour blender ingredients into food processor with dry ingredients and mix until it looks like a soft dough. Spread on counter with more coconut flour and knead until dough is not sticky. Let dough rest for 10-20 minutes.

Use about ¼ cup to form a ball. Flatten balls and make a hole in the middle for bagel shape, or use a donut pan. If using donut pan remove from pan as soon as the shape is formed.

Place on a dehydrator and dry about 2 hours. Cut each bagel in half and continue drying for another 2 or so hours. It is ready when the desired texture is achieved.

Serving suggestion: tastes good with herbed vegan cream cheese (page 148).

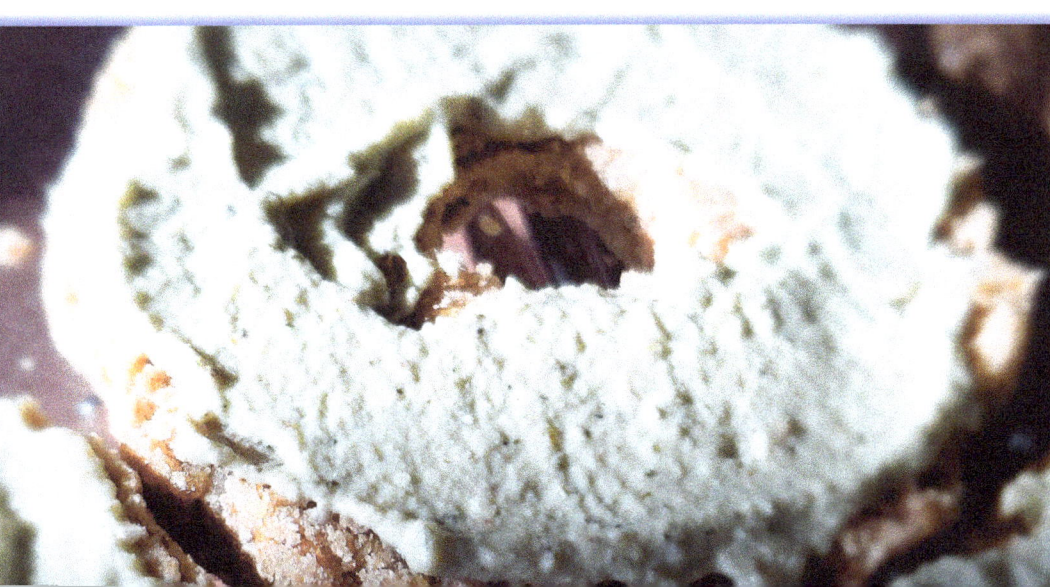

Pizza Crackers

Preparation: 30 Min. Soaking: 8-12 Hrs. Drying: 6-10 Hrs. Makes 6-8 Servings

Ingredients

- 1 c. almonds
- ½ c. pumpkin seeds
- 1 red bell pepper
- 1-2 carrots
- 2-3 stalks celery
- ¼ c. onion
- 1 tsp. parsley
- ½ c. raw tahini
- 2 cloves, garlic
- 1 tsp. basil
- 3 tbsp. pizza seasoning
- 1 tsp. onion powder
- 1 tbsp. Himalayan crystal salt
- 1 tsp. cold pressed olive oil
- pure water as needed

Directions

Soak almonds and pumpkin seeds overnight. Drain water off and place nuts in a food processor.

Cut and seed bell pepper. Slice celery into small pieces and place in food processor along with bell pepper, carrots, parsley, garlic, olive oil, tahini, and spices combine until mixed. And only enough water as needed to achieve desired texture

Spread dough on a nonstick dehydrator sheet it should be about a half an inch thick. Lightly cut into desired shape. Dehydrate at 100°F for about 3 hours. Flip and carefully remove nonstick dehydrator sheet. Continue drying until desired dryness is obtained approximately 4 more hours.

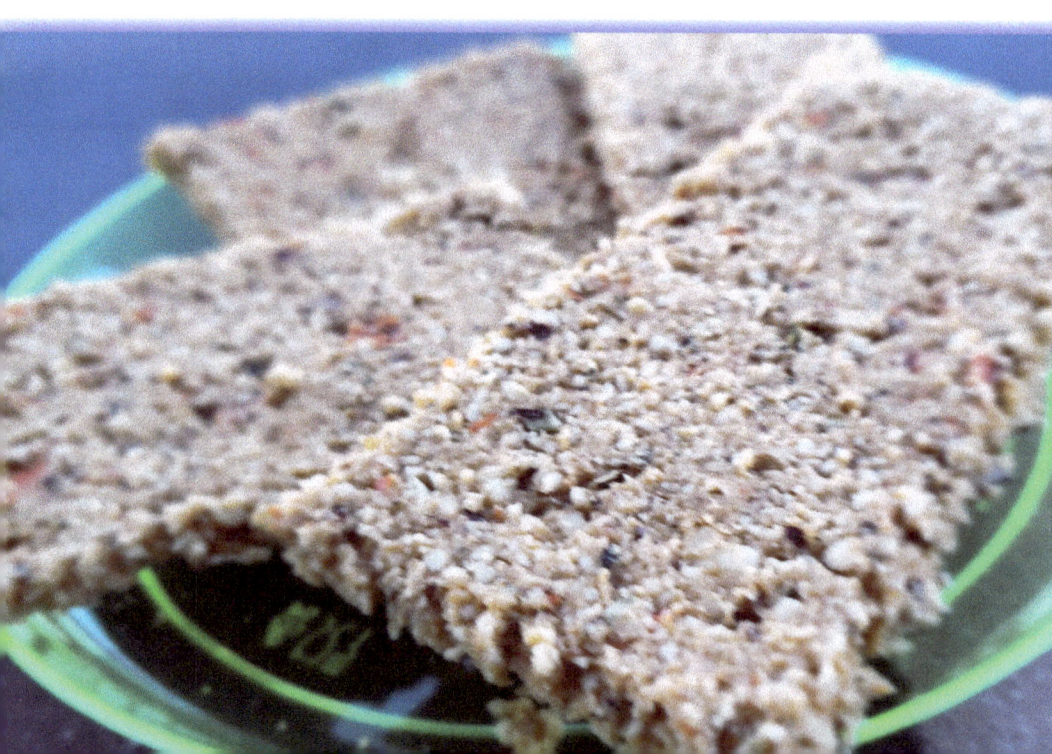

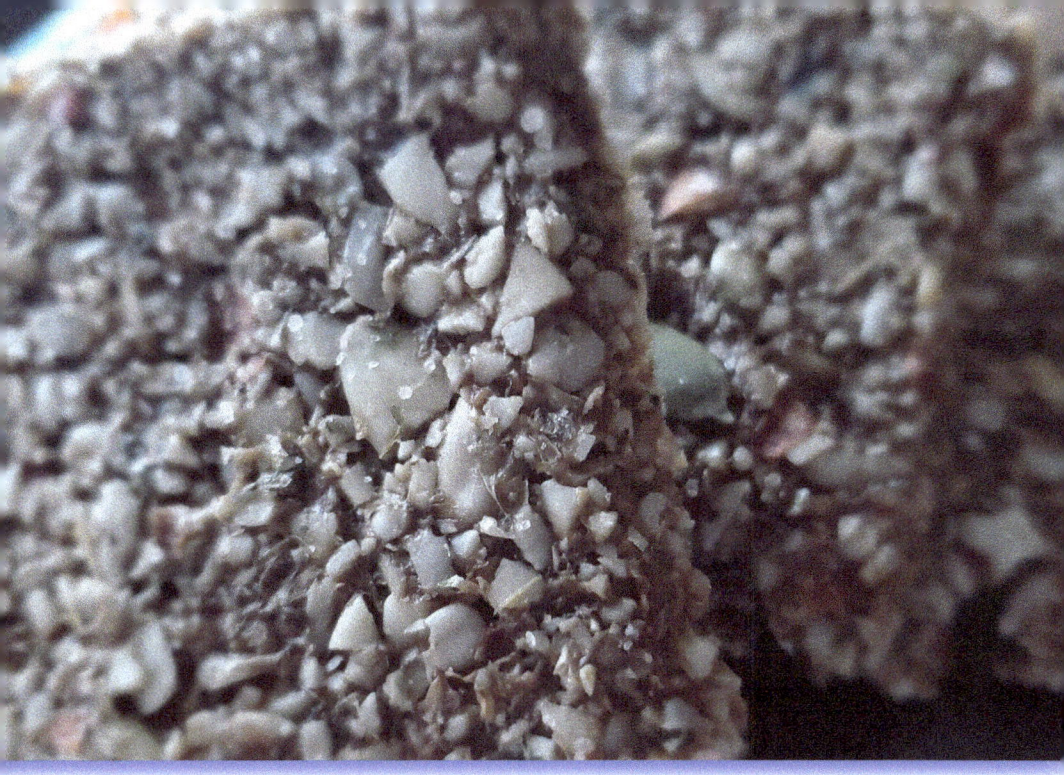

Veggie Crackers

Preparation: 20 Min. | **Soaking:** 8-12 Hrs. | **Drying:** 6-10 Hrs. | **Makes 6-8 Servings**

Ingredients

- 1-2 cloves garlic
- 1 tomato
- 2 carrots
- 1 c. raw sunflower seeds
- 1 c. raw pumpkin seeds
- 1 red bell pepper
- 1 onion
- 3 celery stalks
- 1 tsp. caraway seeds
- 1 tsp. Himalayan crystal salt
- 2 tbsp. cold pressed olive oil
- 3 tbsp. raw tahini

Directions

Soak pumpkin and sunflower seeds overnight, drain water off and place seeds into food processor. Combine seeds and shredded carrots in food processor until finely chopped.

To mixture add tomato, garlic, bell pepper, onion, celery, tahini, olive oil, and salt blend until everything is well incorporated.

Spread onto a nonstick dehydrator sheet about a quarter of an inch thick. Lightly score, the crackers and place in a dehydrator at 100°F for about 4 hours.

Flip crackers and carefully remove nonstick dehydrator sheet. Continue drying until desired crispness is obtained.

Sesame Crackers

Preparation: 30 Min.   Soaking: 8-12 Hrs.   Drying: 12-24 Hrs.   Makes 6-8 Servings

Ingredients

- ½ lemon, juiced
- 1 tsp. cumin
- 1 tsp. curry
- 1 c. sunflower seeds
- 1 c. sesame seeds
- 1 c. carrot pulp
- 1 small red onion

Directions

Soak sesame and sunflower seeds separately overnight. Drain water and rinse then set aside.

In a food processor, combine a half cup sesame seeds, all the sunflower seeds, carrot pulp, onion, lemon juice, cumin, and curry until smooth.

Form dough into balls using 2 teaspoons of batter. Place on a dehydrator tray with a nonstick dehydrator sheet and flatten to a quarter of an inch thick. Sprinkle with remaining sesame seeds.

Dehydrate at 105°F for 2 hours. Flip the crackers and carefully remove the nonstick dehydrator sheet. Continue dehydrating for 4 or more hours until desired crispness is obtained.

Fun Fact

Curry powder is a mixture of spices of widely varying composition. The British developed it after they colonized India to describe a specific mixture of spices, which then became a fixture in British cooking.

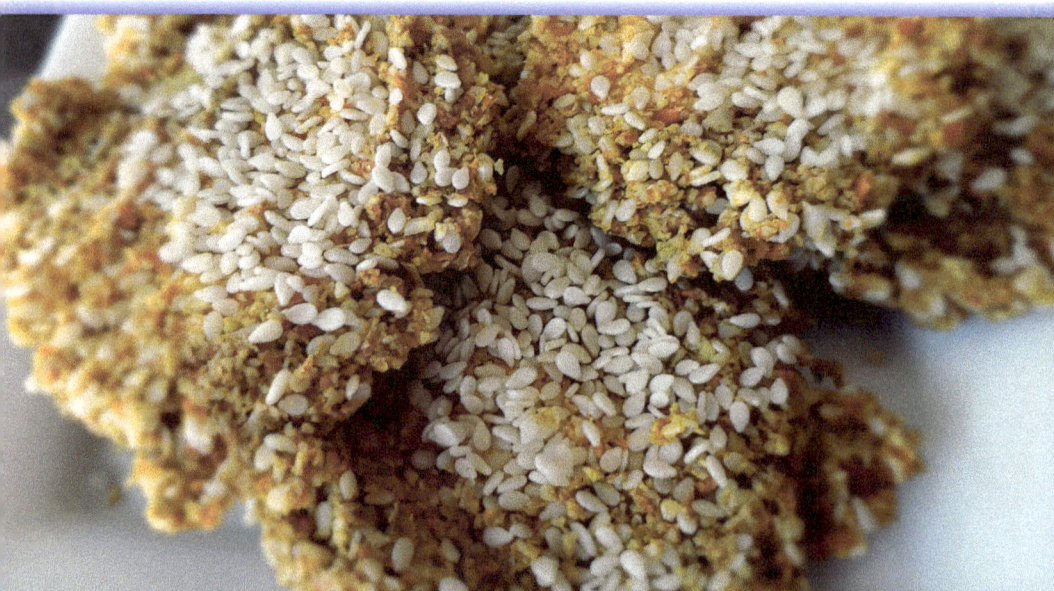

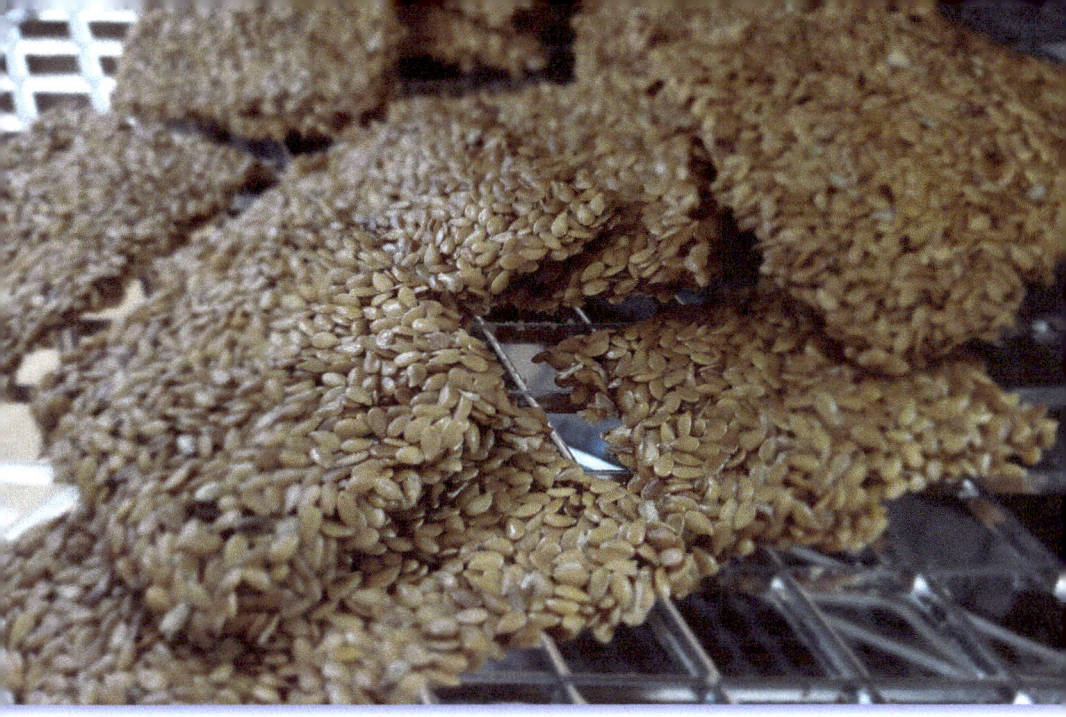

Basic Flaxseed Crackers

Preparation: 30 Min. *Soaking: 8-12 Hrs.* *Drying: 12-24 Hrs.* *Makes 6-8 Servings*

Ingredients

- 1 c. flax seeds
- ¾ c. pure water
- ¼ tsp. Himalayan crystal salt

Directions

Mix flax seeds with salt, pour water over flax and stir well. Let mixture soak 2-4 hours.

Spread mixture thin and evenly on a non-stick dehydrator sheet.

Dry for about 6 hours. Take the crackers out and turn them over and pull off the non-stick sheet. Continue drying for another 6-15 hours or until they are dry.

Variations

For corn flaxseed crackers add corn and soaked buckwheat.

For Italian flaxseed crackers add Italian spices and chopped tomatoes.

Note

There are many ways to make these crackers. If you do not like whole flaxseed, then grind them in a coffee grinder before adding water. Use your imagination and make the flax crackers you enjoy.

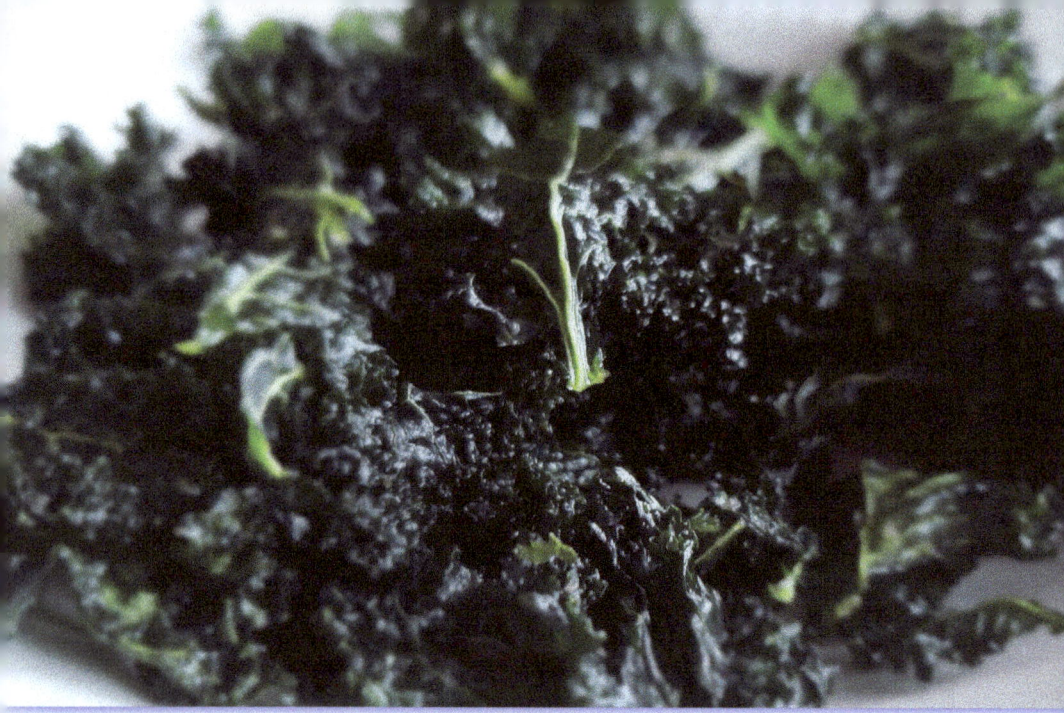

Kale Chips

Preparation: 20 Min. Drying: 8-16 Hrs. Makes 6-8 Servings

Ingredients

- 1 bunch kale
- 1 tbsp. cold pressed olive oil
- 1 tsp. Himalayan crystal salt

Directions

Using a knife or kitchen shears carefully remove leaves from thick stems and tear into large pieces. Wash and thoroughly dry kale.

In a bowl, mix the olive oil and salt. Massage oil mixture into kale.

Place kale on a dehydrator try and dry for half an hour to one hour. Chips should be crispy when done

Note

You can make any flavor of kale chips by adding seasonings.

After massage, the oil into the kale add desired flavor.

Fun Fact

Eating kale with fatty foods, like avocado or olive oil, makes it easier for your body to absorb some of the nutrients kale has to offer.

Broccoli Crunchy

Preparation: 20 Min. Drying: 8-16 Hrs. Makes 6-8 Servings

Ingredients

- 3 pounds broccoli florets
- 2 ½ c. cashew mayo (page 143)

Directions

Make cashew mayo and set aside. Wash and cut broccoli into small pieces.

Place broccoli and mayo in a bowl. Mix making sure the broccoli is very well coated you may need to add more mayo.

Place on dehydrator trays and dry and 115°F for about 8-16 hours or until completely dry.

Variations

For a cheesy broccoli only dry for half the time or until broccoli is soft.

Fun Fact

As early as May of 1767 Thomas Jefferson, one of the founding fathers of the United States, imported broccoli seeds from Italy to plant at Monticello.

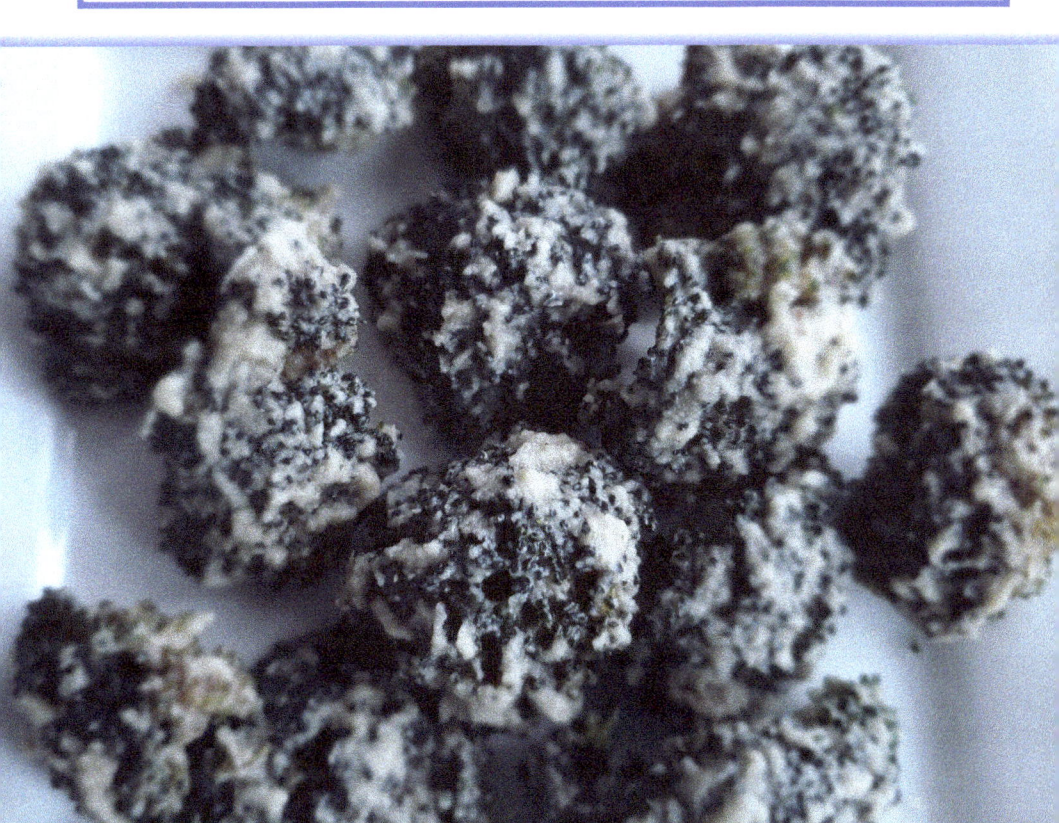

Almond Milk

Preparation: *Soaking:*   *Makes 6-8*
5 Min.   *8-12 Hrs.*   *Servings*

Ingredients

- 1 c. almonds, soaked
- 2 c. pure water

Note

For a whiter milk peel of brown skin before blending. Save almond pulp for use in another recipe such as almond mayo, cookies, crackers, or bread.

Other nuts that are good for nut milks include pumpkin seeds, hazelnuts, Brazil nuts, sesame seeds, hemp seeds, walnut, and pecan.

To make replace almonds with chosen nut or seed.

Directions

Cover almonds with water and soak overnight, drain off water and place nuts into a blender with 2 cups fresh water. Blend for a minute or two.

Using a milk bag, (clean nylon sock, or cheesecloth) over a big bowl, pour contents of the blender into bag. Then squeeze out liquid for milk. Sweeten milk if desired.

> ### Fun Fact
>
> *Almond milk contains no saturated fat or dietary cholesterol.*

Coconut Cream

Preparation: *Makes 6-8*
15 Min.   *Servings*

Ingredients

- 1 young coconut
- coconut water
- 2 tbsp. raw coconut nectar
- ¼ inch vanilla bean or raw vanilla powder

> ### Fun Fact
>
> *Research is being done to see if coconut can be used in hair regrowth and anti-aging cosmetics.*

Directions

Open young coconut, reserve the water for use later. Scrape out coconut meat and place it in a blender with vanilla and coconut nectar.

Blend until nice and fluffy slowly adding coconut water in order to achieve fluffiness.

Drink any leftover coconut water.

Cashew Cream

Preparation: *Makes 6-8*
10 Min.   *Servings*

Ingredients

- 2 c. cashews
- 1 ½ c. pure water
- ½ c. raw liquid sweetener
- ¼ inch vanilla bean or raw vanilla powder

Directions

In a blender, combine cashew nuts, orange juice, agave nectar, and vanilla. Add just enough water to achieve a very creamy texture.

Almond Mayo

Preparation: *Soaking:*   *Makes 6-8*
10 Min.   *8-12 Hrs.*   *Servings*

Ingredients

- 2 c. almonds, soaked
- 3 tbsp. onion or 1 tbsp. onion powder
- ½ c. cold pressed olive oil
- ¾ c. pure water
- 1-2 tbsp. Himalayan crystal salt
- ½ lemon, juiced

Directions

Soak almonds overnight, drain water off. Peel brown shell off almond, while they are wet.

Place the peeled almonds into a blender, add olive oil, onion powder, salt, and lemon juice and blend until creamy.

Slowly add water until a creamy mayo consistency is achieved

> **Fun Fact**
>
> *Almonds are mentioned in the Old Testament of the Bible. See Genesis 43:11*

Variation

1) For cashew mayo substitute cashew nuts for almonds. Cashews can become rubbery so I usually do not soak them very long if at all.

Almond Sour Cream

Preparation: 15 Min. *Soaking:* 8-12 Hrs. *Makes 6-8 Servings*

Ingredients

- 1 c. almonds, soaked
- 1 tsp. lemon Juice
- 1 tbsp. raw apple cider vinegar
- ½ c. pure water as needed
- Himalayan crystal salt

Directions

Soak almonds overnight, drain water off. While almonds are still wet, peel off brown skin. If the skin is left, you will have a brown flaked sour cream.

In a blender, combine peeled almonds, lemon juice, raw apple cider vinegar, and salt purée add only enough water to make it creamy.

Taste and adjust seasoning; you may need more lemon or vinegar if it's not sour enough.

Fun Fact

In raw apple cider vinegar, the mother has not been filter out. Mother is the murky or cobweb like stuff that is in the bottom of unfiltered vinegar.

Nancy's Peruvian Cheese

Preparation: 20 Min. *Soaking:* 8-12 Hrs. *Drying:* 8-12 Hrs. *Makes 6-8 Servings*

Ingredients

- 1 c. basic cheese (page 145)
- ½ c. cold pressed olive oil
- 3 Anaheim peppers, seeded
- 2 cloves garlic
- ½ small onion
- ¼ - ½ c. almonds
- 1 tsp. curry
- 1 lemon, juiced
- Himalayan crystal salt
- ¼ - ½ c. nut milk (page 142)

Directions

Make basic cheese and soak almonds overnight.

Place cheese, olive oil, garlic, onion, almonds, curry, lemon juice, salt, and seeded Anaheim peppers into a blender, slowly add milk until a smooth texture is achieved.

Serving suggestion: Place lettuce on a plate. Shred sweet potato or jicama onto the plate, layer sprouts over the top and garnish with tomatoes and sundried olives.

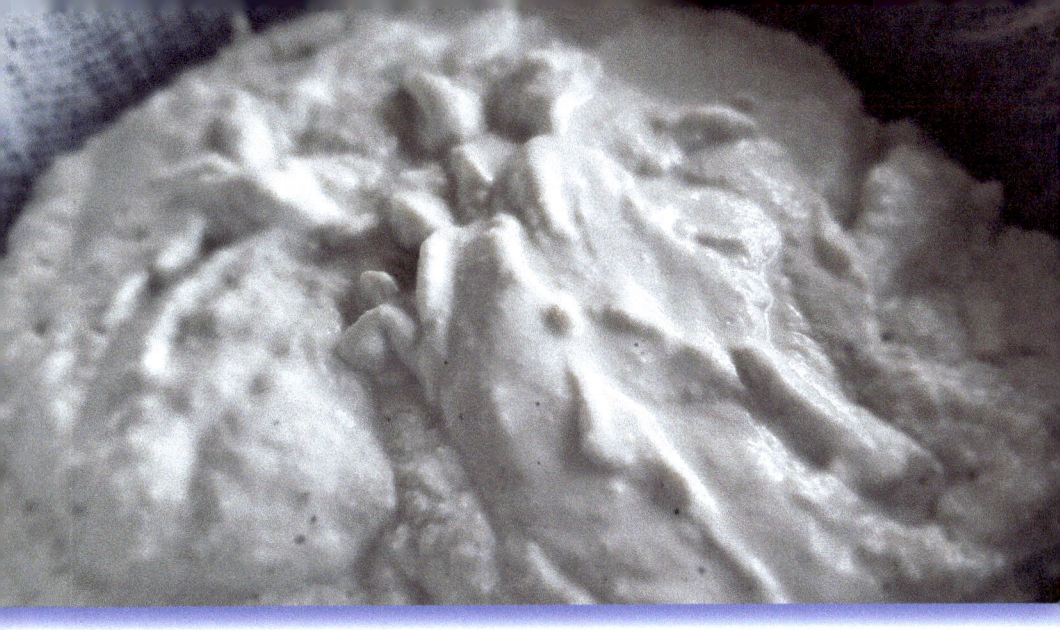

Basic Seed Cheese

Preparation: 35 Min. Soaking: 8-12 Hrs. Fermenting: 12-18 Hrs. Makes 6-8 Servings

Ingredients

- 1 c. sunflower seeds
- 1 c. pumpkin seeds
- 1 c. rejuvelac

Directions

Soak pumpkin and sunflower seeds overnight, drain off water and set aside.

Pour rejuvelac and half the seeds into a blender, blend at high speed until well blended. Add remaining seeds to the blender and combine until it is a smooth thick paste about 4 minutes.

Pour mixture into cheese cloth and place in a bowl or jar cover with a clean towel or cloth, and leave it for 8-12 hours. The longer it stands, the stronger the flavor will be.

After fermentation time elapses, discard liquid that has settled at the bottom of the jar. Store extra cheese in refrigerator; cover tightly.

Variations

1) May replace the rejuvelac with the juice of 1 lemon, 1 tablespoon. raw apple cider vinegar and 1 cup pure water

2) Try making this cheese with almonds. Combinations of almonds, sunflower seeds, and sesame are also very flavorful.

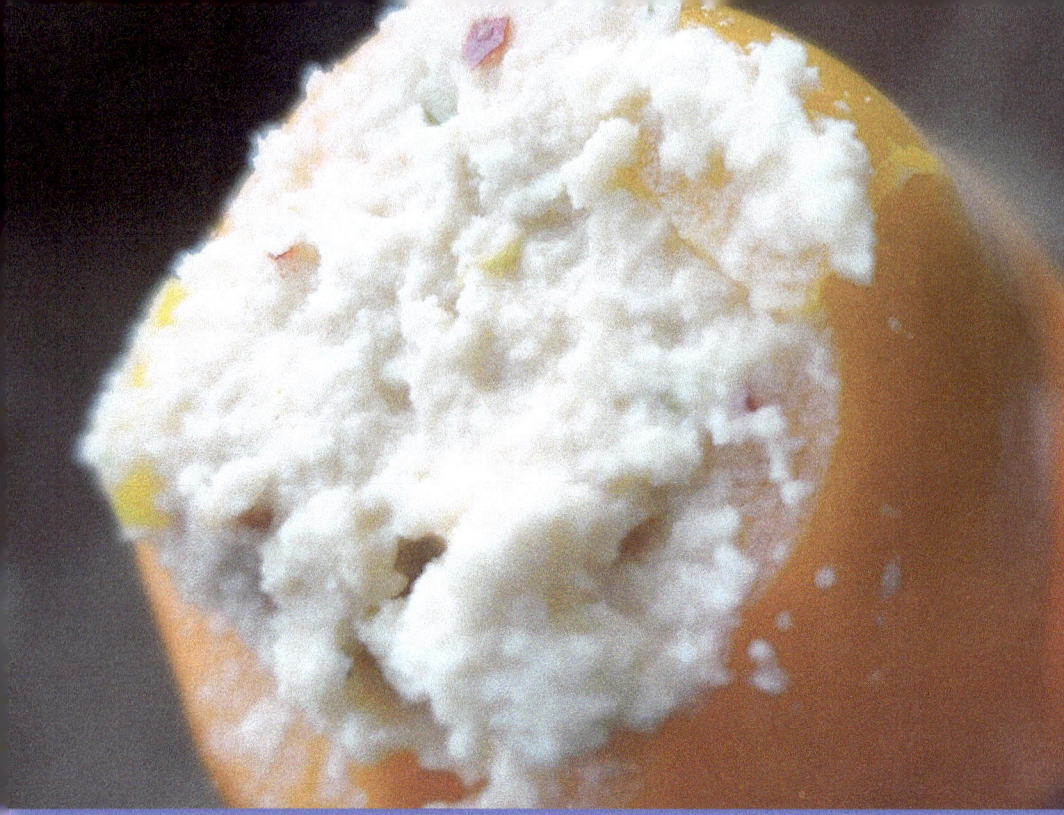

Spicy Cheese

Preparation: 15 Min. Soaking: 8-12 Hrs. Makes 6-8 Servings

Ingredients

- 2 c. almonds, soaked
- ½ c. lemon, juiced
- ½ tsp. Himalayan crystal salt
- 1 tsp. dill
- ½ c. green onion, chopped
- 1 red bell pepper, diced
- 1 chili pepper
- ½ c. dried tomatoes
- ¼ c. cold pressed olive oil

Directions

Soak almonds overnight. Drain water off almonds. Save soaking water from tomatoes to use if needed but don't use the almond water.

In a small bowl, place dried tomatoes and olive oil and let soak for 30 min. You can use fresh tomatoes if available.

In a food processor, place almonds, lemon juice, salt, dill, green onion, red bell pepper, and chili pepper, process until well mixed. Place in a bowl incorporate tomatoes and mix with a spoon. Chill and serve.

Serving suggestion; serve on a flax cracker or other raw cracker, as a dip with vegetables or stuffed in mini bell peppers.

Honey Butter

Preparation: *Soaking:*   *Makes 6-8*
10 Min.   *8-12 Hrs.*   *Servings*

Ingredients

- ½ c. coconut oil
- 4 tbsp. raw honey or other raw liquid sweetener
- ¼ tsp. turmeric
- 1 tsp. Himalayan crystal salt

Directions

In a small bowl, whip coconut oil by hand. Add honey, turmeric, and salt; continue beating by hand until nice and fluffy and well mixed.

Serving suggestion: Tastes really good on the cornbread (page 132).

Gourmet Garlic Butter

Preparation: *Soaking:*   *Makes 6-8*
10 Min.   *8-12 Hrs.*   *Servings*

Ingredients

- ½ c. coconut oil
- 1-2 cloves garlic
- pinch basil leaves
- pinch dill
- pinch Himalayan crystal salt
- pinch of nutritional yeast (optional)

Directions

In a bowl, combine coconut oil, minced garlic, dill, salt, nutritional yeast and basil mix until well combined.

Serving suggestion; spread on Nancy's bread for garlic bread.

Rawmesan

Preparation: *Soaking:*   *Makes 6-8*
10 Min.   *8-12 Hrs.*   *Servings*

Ingredients

- ½ c. cashews
- ¼ c. raw, pumpkin seeds
- ½ tsp. Himalayan crystal salt
- ½ tsp. dill
- ½ tsp. nutritional yeast (optional)

Directions

In a food processor, grind dry cashews and dry pumpkin seed into a powder. Add salt, dill, and nutritional yeast pulse a few more times.

Rawmesan will keep about a month in the refrigerator.

Vegan Fruit Cream Cheese

Preparation: 20 Min. *Soaking:* 2-12 Hrs. *Makes 6-8 Servings*

Ingredients

- ½ c. cashews
- ½ c. macadamia nuts
- 1 lemons, juiced
- ½ tsp. Himalayan crystal salt
- ½ c. fresh fruit (strawberries, raspberry, pineapple, blueberry or other fruit)
- 1 tbsp. coconut oil
- ¼ c. rejuvelac or water

Directions

Soak cashews and macadamia nuts for 10 minutes. Drain off water and place nuts into a food processor add lemon juice and mix until smooth

Wash fruit and place in food processor with nuts, mix until desired texture is achieved. This can be big chunks or very smooth.

Variation

For plain cream cheese omit fruit.

Herbed Cream Cheese

Preparation: 20 Min. *Soaking:* 2-12 Hrs. *Makes 6-8 Servings*

Ingredients

- ½ c. cashews
- ½ c. pumpkin seeds
- 2 lemons, juiced
- ½ tsp. Himalayan crystal salt
- ¼ tsp. nutritional yeast (optional)
- ½ tsp. chives
- ½ tsp. dried oregano
- ½ tsp. dried parsley
- ½ tsp. dried basil
- ¼ tsp. dried dill

Directions

Soak pumpkin seeds overnight. Drain off water and add to food processor.

Soak the cashews for 10 minutes. Drain off water and add to pumpkin seeds.

Juice lemons and add the juice to food processor add salt, nutritional yeast, chives oregano, parsley, basil, and dill then process until smooth. Add water a tablespoon at a time to thin mixture if needed.

Place in a dish and cover. Chill for about an hour or until ready to serve. Can store in a sealed container for 4-7 days.

Vegan Feta Cheese

Preparation:	Soaking:	Fermenting:	Makes 6-8
20 Min.	8-12 Hrs.	8-18 Hrs.	Servings

Ingredients

- 1 c. almonds
- ¼ c. fresh basil or thyme oregano or other spice
- ¼ tsp. Himalayan crystal salt
- ½ c. rejuvalic

Directions

Soak almonds overnight drain the water off. Peel brown skin off almonds while wet.

Pour rejuvelac into a blender with almonds and salt. Blend at high speed, until it is smooth.

Chop fresh basil and pulse into the cheese mixture or mix by hand. If using the blender make sure that it only pulsed otherwise you will have a green cheese.

Pour blender mixture into cheese cloth over a bowl or glass jar. Wrap the edges of the cloth and gently squeezing the liquid out. Hang cloth ball over the bowl, and leave it for 8-12 hours. The longer it stands the stronger the flavor will be.

After fermentation, time elapses, discard any liquid that has settle on bottom of bowl or jar. Store extra cheese in refrigerator; covered tightly.

Variation

If you don't have rejuvelac, you can use lemon, and a half a cup of water instead. If you use this method, however, the fermentation time may need to be extended to 12 -18 hours.

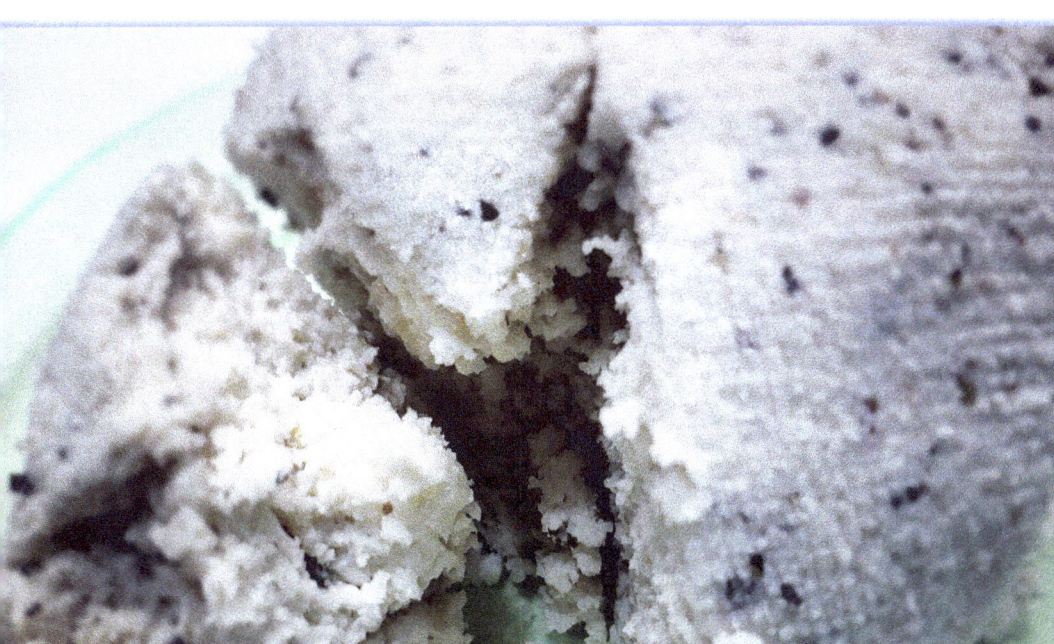

Irish Moss Gel

Preparation: *Soaking:*   *Makes 6-8*
15 Min.   *8-12 Hrs.*   *Servings*

Ingredients

- 1 c. Irish moss
- 2-3 c. pure water

Directions

Rinse Irish moss. Soak in water for 30 minutes. Drain and rinse again make sure the moss is clean then soak overnight in a glass jar, then drain.

Place Irish moss in a blender with just enough fresh water to cover. Blend until smooth, it may take a few minutes.

Pour into a clean jar with a lid. Store in refrigerator up to 3 weeks.

Fun Fact

Irish Moss is a tough and stringy seaweed that grows on rocks in tidal pools along the northern Atlantic. It is a thickening agent for jellies, puddings, and soups, and is a traditional herbal remedy in Ireland.

The human body is made up of 102 minerals and Irish Moss contains 92 of them. It also provides a wealth of other important nutrients including; protein, beta-carotene, B vitamins, pectin, and vitamin C.

Brother John's Tabasco

Preparation: *Soaking:*   *Makes 1*
15 Min.   *8-12 Hrs.*   *Cup*

Ingredients

- 3 red bell peppers
- 2 tbsp. raw apple cider vinegar
- 1 red hot (serrano or jalapeno) pepper
- ½ c. water or more as needed
- 2 tbsp. lime, juiced
- ¼ c. onion
- ½ tsp. Himalayan crystal salt
- ½ tsp. white pepper
- ¼ tsp. paprika

Directions

Cut and seed peppers, place into a blender with vinegar, lime juice, onion, salt pepper, and paprika. Purée and until smooth adding water to achieve desired texture.

Note

If you want fire hot tabasco leave seeds in the hot pepper.

Ketchup

Preparation: 10 Min. *Soaking: 1-3 Hrs.* *Makes ½ Cup*

Ingredients

- ½ c. dried tomatoes, soaked
- 2 fresh tomatoes
- ¼ c. raw apple cider vinegar
- 3 tbsp. onion
- 1 clove garlic
- 1 tbsp. Himalayan crystal salt

Directions

Soak the dried tomatoes in water for 2 hours. Remove tomatoes from water and place in a blender.

To the blender, add fresh tomatoes, vinegar, onion, garlic, and salt purée until well blended.

Arugula Pesto

Preparation: 20 Min. *Soaking: 8-12 Hrs.* *Makes 2 Cups*

Ingredients

- ½ c. sunflower seeds, soaked
- ½ c. pumpkin seeds, soaked
- 4 c. arugula, stems removed
- 6 tbsp. cold pressed olive oil
- 1 lemon, juiced
- 2 cloves garlic
- black pepper to taste

Directions

Soak pumpkin and sunflower seeds overnight. Drain off water and place seeds in a food processor.

Remove thick stems from arugula and place in food processor add olive oil, lemon juice, garlic, salt, and pepper. Process until well combined.

Almond Butter

Preparation: 40 Min. *Makes 2 Cup*

Ingredients

- 2 c. raw almonds
- 3 tbsp. cold pressed olive oil
- ½ tsp. Himalayan crystal salt (optional)

Directions

Place dry almonds in food processor and grind into a fine powder. Continue to process until the nuts make a ball then begins to smooth out it will take a long time to get to a smooth constancy. May need to rest food processor before almonds smooth out.

Add oil a tablespoon at a time. Until desired constancy is achieved. You may need more or less oil to achieve the constancy you like.

Note

Don't use water as it will make the mixture seized and ruin almond butter.

Tahini Sauce

Preparation: *Soaking:*   *Makes 1*
20 Min.   *8-12 Hrs.*   *Cup*

Ingredients

- 1 small onion
- 1 tbsp. cold pressed olive oil
- 1 c. raw tahini
- ¾ c. pure water
- 2-3 cloves garlic
- 1 lemon, juiced
- dash cumin
- Himalayan crystal salt
- black pepper to taste
- bunch of parsley

Directions

Blend onion, olive oil, tahini, water, garlic, lemon juice, cumin salt and pepper in a blender until smooth. Garnish with chopped parsley.

Fun Fact

According to the historian Herodotus sesame was cultivated 3500 years ago in Ancient Iraq.

Tahini

Preparation: *Soaking:*   *Makes 1*
20 Min.   *8-12 Hrs.*   *Cup*

Ingredients

- ¾ c. sesame seeds
- 2 tbsp. cold pressed olive oil
- 1 tsp. Himalayan crystal salt
- 1 lemon, juiced
- ¼ c. water

Directions

Grind sesame seeds in a coffee grinder to make sesame flour and place in a bowl.

Add salt and lemon juice to flour and mix. Gradually add oil until desired consistency is achieved.

Stores in the fridge up to one month.

Fun Facts

Tahini is the result of ground sesames seeds blended into a paste or butter.

Sesame is grown primarily for its oil rich seeds; which come in a variety of colors, from cream to black. Heating damages the healthy polyunsaturated fats.

Seasonal Vegetable Chart

Arugula	Spring, Summer, Fall
Asparagus	Spring
Avocadoes	Spring, Summer, Fall, Winter
Basil	Spring, Summer
Beans	Spring, Summer, Fall, Winter
Beets	Spring, Summer, Fall, Winter
Broccoli	Spring, Summer, Fall, Winter
Brussels Sprouts	Fall, Winter
Burdock	Summer, Fall
Cabbage	Spring, Summer, Fall, Winter
Carrots	Spring, Summer, Fall, Winter
Cauliflower	Spring, Fall, Winter
Celery	Spring, Summer, Fall
Chard	Spring, Summer, Fall, Winter
Collards	Summer, Fall, Winter
Corn	Summer, Fall
Cucumbers	Spring, Summer, Fall
Eggplant	Spring, Summer, Fall
Fennel	Spring, Summer, Fall, Winter
Garlic	Spring, Summer, Fall, Winter
Herbs	Spring, Summer, Fall, Winter
Kale	Spring, Summer, Fall, Winter
Leeks	Spring, Summer, Fall, Winter
Lettuces	Spring, Summer, Fall, Winter
Mushrooms	Spring, Summer, Fall, Winter
Onions	Spring, Summer, Fall, Winter
Parsnips	Fall, Winter
Peas	Spring, Summer, Fall
Peppers, Bell	Spring, Summer, Fall
Peppers, Chili	Spring, Summer, Fall
Radish	Spring, Summer, Fall, Winter
Rhubarb	Spring, Summer, Fall
Rutabaga	Fall, Winter
Spinach	Spring, Summer, Fall, Winter

Squash, Summer	Summer
Squash, Winter	Winter
Sunchokes (Jerusalem Artichokes)	Fall, Winter
Sweet Potatoes	Fall, Winter
Tomatoes	Spring, Fall, Winter
Turnips	Fall, Winter

Seasonal Fruit Chart

Apples	Fall
Apricots	Spring
Asian Pears	Summer, Fall
Blackberries	Spring
Blueberries	Spring
Boysenberries	Spring
Cherries	Spring
Dates	Fall
Dates, Dried	Spring, Summer, Fall, Winter
Figs	Summer, Fall
Grapefruit	Fall, Winter
Grapes	Summer, Fall
Kiwi	Fall, Winter
Lemons	Spring, Summer, Fall, Winter
Limes	Summer, Fall, Winter
Melons	Summer, Fall
Mulberries	Summer
Oranges	Spring, Summer, Fall, Winter
Peaches	Summer, Fall
Pears	Fall
Plums	Spring, Summer
Pomegranates	Fall, Winter
Raspberries	Spring, Summer, Fa
Strawberries	Spring, Summer
Tangerines	Winter

Index

A

Almond Butter 151
Almond Delight 86
Almond Mayo 143
Almond Milk 142
Almond Sour Cream 144
Anytime Breakfast Burrito 80
Apple Carrot Muffins 131
Apple Curry Rice 69
Apple Pie 106
Arugula Pesto 151

B

Baja Pulled Eggplant Burrito 90
Baja Sauce 90
Banana Date Kebabs 129
Bar Desserts
  Black Bottom Coconut Bars 113
  Blond Ambition 114
  Carrot Brownies 116
  Lemon Bars 117
  Peanut Butter Bars 115
Basic Flaxseed Crackers 139
Basic Pâté 57
Basic Seed Cheese 145
Basil Citrus Juice 22
Baykon 87
Bean Burrito 75
Beet Hummus 54
Berry Tall Cake 99
Beverage
  Almond Milk 142
  Basil Citrus Juice 22
  Chamomile Lemonade 16
  Frosty Drink 19
  Hazelnut Drink 23
  Hibiscus Drink 17
  Mango Smoothie 18
  Mexican Mind Meld 21
  Mint Shake 18
  Peach Mint Lemonade 20
  Rejuvelac 24
  Snapin Carrot Juice 22
  Strawberry Frosty 19
  Tabbouleh Smoothie 24

  Watermelon Strawberry Drink 25
Blackberry Torte 109
Black Bottom Coconut Bars 113
Blond Ambition 114
Brazil Nut Burger 74
Bread
  Apple Carrot Muffins 131
  Cinnamon Rolls 112
  Corn Bread 132
  Garlic Bread. 147
  Hazelnut Bagels 135
  Lemon Poppy Muffins 130
  Nancy's Bread 134
  Rye Bread 133
Broccoli Crunchy 141
Broccoli Soup 32
Brother John's Tabasco 150
Brussels Sprout Hazelnut Salad 49
Buckwheat
  Apple Carrot Muffins 131
  Celebration Cake 101
  Corn Flaxseed Crackers 139
  Impossible Zucchini Pie 97
  Mediterranean Buckwheat Salad 47
  Moroccan Buckwheat Salad 40
  Nancy's Bread 134
  Rye Bread 133
  Soft Gingerbread Cookies 128
Buttered Zucchini 93

C

Cabbage
  Sauerkraut 60
  Stuffed Tomato with Cabbage Salad 46
Cake
  Berry Tall Cake 99
  Celebration Cake 101
  German Chocolate Cake 100
  Pumpkin Cake 103
  Pumpkin Cheesecake 105
  Raspberry Lemon Cake 102
  Sweet Kale Cheesecake 104
Candied Kale 110
Carob 120
Carob Frosting 99

Carrot Brownies 116
Carrot Ginger Cookies 127
Carrot Hummus 56
Carrot Mushroom Stir-fry 59
Carrot Raisin Salad 37
Cashew Cream 143
Cashew Milk 142
Cauliflower
   Cauliflower Tacos 95
   Cauliflower Wings 81
   Pickled Cauliflower 61
   Smart Cat Salad 35
Cauliflower Tacos 95
Cauliflower Wings 81
Celebration Cake 101
Chamomile Lemonade 16
Cheese Sauce 76
Cheesy Broccoli 141
Cherry Dressing 51
Chocolate Cherry Pie 122
Chocolate Dipped Ice Cream Sandwich 120
Chocolate Ice Cream 119
Cinnamon Rolls 112
Coconut Cream 142
Coconut Sugar Bumps 110
Collard Herb Rolls 71
Cool Cucumber Soup 28
Corn Bread 132
Corn Flaxseed Crackers 139
Crackers
   Basic Flaxseed Crackers 139
   Corn Flaxseed Crackers 139
   Italian Flaxseed Crackers 139
   Pizza Crackers 136
Cravin' Mac & Cheese 79
Cream Cheese 148
Cream Frosting 110
Creamy Lemon Poppy Seed Dressing 51
Curry Powder 138

D

Dairy
   Almond Mayo 143
   Almond Milk 142
   Almond Sour Cream 144
   Basic Seed Cheese 145
   Cashew Cream 143
   Cashew Milk 142
   Cheese Sauce 76
   Coconut Cream 142
   Cream Cheese 148
   Gourmet Garlic Butter 147
   Hazel Nut Milk 142
   Hemp Seed Milk 142
   Herbed Cream Cheese 148
   Honey Butter 147
   Nancy's Peruvian Cheese 144
   Rawmesan 147
   Sesame Seed Milk 142
   Spicy Cheese 146
   Vegan Feta Cheese 149
   Vegan Fruit Cream Cheese 148
Dirty Rice 69
Drying Nuts & Seeds 14

E

Eggless Salad 34
Eggless Salad Sandwich 71
Eggplant
   Baja Pulled Eggplant Burrito 90
   Baykon 87
   Eggplant Kebabs 96
   Middle Eastern Marinated Eggplant 78
   Pulled Eggplant 90
Eggplant Kebabs 96

F

Falafel Patties 37
Falafel Salad 36
Fiesta Salad 39
Flax Balls 111
Flaxseed Crackers 139
Flora's Albanian Salad 44
Frosty Drink 19
Frozen Desserts
   Chocolate Dipped Ice Cream Sandwich 120
   Chocolate Ice Cream 119
   Fudge Sickle 114
   Stawberry Ice Cream 118
Fruit Cream Cheese 148
Fudge 129
Fudge Sickle 114

G

Garlic Bread. 147
Garlic Butter 147

German Chocolate Cake 100
German Chocolate Donuts 100
Gingerbread Cookies 128
Gourmet Garlic Butter 147
Greek Dressing 50
Greek Salad 50
Green Zoodles 92
Ground Meatless 57
Guacamole 59

H

Hazelnut Bagels 135
Hazelnut Drink 23
Hazel Nut Milk 142
Hemp Seed Milk 142
Herbed Almond Spread 58
Herbed Cream Cheese 148
Hibiscus Drink 17
Honey Butter 147
How to sprout garbanzo beans 35

I

Impossible Zucchini Pie 97
Introducing the family 10
Irish Moss Gel 150
Italian Dressing 52
Italian Flaxseed Crackers 139

J

Jalapeño Poppers 66

K

Kale Chips 140
Kale Hummus 55
Kale Strawberry Salad 43
Ketchup 151

L

Lasagna 76
Lemon Bars 117
Lemon Pie 108
Lemon Poppy Muffins 130
Lemon Rice 67
Lovage 34

M

Mango Smoothie 18

Marinara Sauce 76
Mayo 143
Mediterranean Buckwheat Salad 47
Mexican Mind Meld 21
Mexican Vegetable Soup 33
Middle Eastern Marinated Eggplant 78
Mint Brownies 116
Mint Shake 18
Mississippi Mud Pie 124
Mom's Apple Pie 106
Moroccan Buckwheat Salad 40
Milk 142

N

Nadhirrah's Jalapeño Poppers 66
Nancy's Bread 134
Nancy's Peruvian Cheese 144
Nut milk 142
Nutty Pumpkin Balls 94

O

Old Fashioned "Potato" Salad 41
Olive Oil 15
Olive Oil Labeling 15
Onion Dip 54
Open Face Tomato Bites 70

P

Parsnip Chowder 27
Party Dip 53
Pâté 57
Peach Mint Lemonade 20
Peach Pie 107
Peanut Butter Bars 115
Peppers 66
Pesto 92, 108, 114
Philly Wrap 73
Pie
  Chocolate Pie 122
  Lemon Pie 108
  Mom's Apple Pie 106
  Peach Pie 107
  Strawberry Pie 123
Pizza Bites 83
Pizza Crackers 136
Pulled Eggplant 90
Pumpkin African Stew 29
Pumpkin Candy 125

Pumpkin Parfait 126
Purple Ribbon 85

R

Raspberry Lemon Cake 102
Rawmesan 147
Rejuvelac 24
Rice
  Apple Curry Rice 69
  Dirty Rice 69
  Lemon Rice 67
  Sprouting Rice 13
  Warm Mexi-Rice 70
  Wild Jambalaya 68
Rye Bread 133

S

Salad
  Brussels Sprout Hazelnut Salad 49
  Carrot Raisin Salad 37
  Eggless Salad 34
  Falafel Salad 36
  Fiesta Salad 39
  Flora's Albanian Salad 44
  Greek Salad 50
  Kale Strawberry Salad 43
  Mediterranean Buckwheat Salad 47
  Moroccan Buckwheat Salad 40
  Old Fashioned "Potato" Salad 41
  Scrambled Corn Salad 45
  Smart Cat Salad 35
  Sprouted Kamut Salad pwith Vinaigrette 42
  Strawberry Kiwi Salad 50
  Stuffed Tomato with Cabbage Salad 46
  Taco Salad 39
  "Tuna" Salad 48
Salad Dressing
  Cherry Dressing 51
  Creamy Lemon Poppy Seed Dressing 51
  Greek Dressing 50
  Italian Dressing 52
  Strawberry Dressing 51
  Tahini Dressing 36
  Tangy Tomato Dressing 52
  Vinaigrette 42
Salsa 59
Salt 14

Samosa 84
Sauerkraut 60
Scrambled Corn Salad 45
Sesame
  Blond Ambition 114
  Carrot Hummus 56
  Eggless Salad 34
  Kale Hummus 55
  Mango Smoothie 18
  Sesame Crackers 138
  Stuffed 'Eggs' 92
  Tahini 152
  Tahini Sauce 152
Sesame Crackers 138
Sesame Seed Milk 142
Shepherd's Pie 88
Simple Salsa 53
Smart Cat Salad 35
Snapin Carrot Juice 22
Snappy Vegetables 63
Soft Gingerbread Cookies 128
Soup
  Broccoli Soup 32
  Cool Cucumber Soup 28
  Mexican Vegetable Soup 33
  Parsnip Chowder 27
  Pumpkin African Stew 29
  Sweet Summer Soup 26
  Vegetable "Noodle" Soup 31
  Vegetable Soup Base 31
Sour Cream 144
Spicy Cheese 146
Spicy Jicama Fries 64
Sprouted Kamut Salad with Vinaigrette 42
Sprouting 13
Sprouting Rice 13
Stawberry Ice Cream 118
Strawberry Dressing 51
Strawberry Frosty 19
Strawberry Kiwi Salad 50
Strawberry Pie 123
Stuffed Anaheim Peppers 65
Stuffed 'Eggs' 92
Stuffed Tomato with Cabbage Salad 46
Sunflower Beans 56
Supplying the Kitchen 11
Sweet Kale Cheesecake 104
Sweet Summer Soup 26

T

Tabbouleh Smoothie 24
Taco Meat 57
Taco Salad 39
Tahini 152
Tahini Dressing 36
Tahini Sauce 152
Tangy Tomato Dressing 52
Tuna Salad 48

V

Vegan Feta Cheese 149
Vegan Fruit Cream Cheese 148
Vegetable "Noodle" Soup 31
Vegetable Pocket 84
Vegetable Soup Base 31
Veggie Crackers 137
Vinaigrette 42

W

Warm Mexi-Rice 70
Watermelon Strawberry Drink 25
Wild Jambalaya 68

Z

Zucchini
   Almond Delight 86
   Buttered Zucchini 93
   Green Zoodles 92
   Hazelnut Bagels 135
   Impossible Zucchini Pie 97
   Lasagna 76
   Mexican Vegetable Soup 33
   Snappy Vegetables 63
   Sweet Kale Cheesecake 104
   "Tuna" Salad 48
   Vegetable "Noodle" Soup 31

Spring Recipe Index

Almond Mayo 143
Almond Milk 142
Almond Sour Cream 144
Anytime Breakfast Burrito 80
Arugula Pesto 151
Banana Date Kebabs 129
Basic Seed Cheese 145
Beet Hummus 54
Berry Tall Cake 99
Blackberry Torte 109
Black Bottom Coconut Bars 113
Blond Ambition 114
Broccoli Soup 32
Candied Kale 110
Carrot Brownies 116
Carrot Ginger Cookies 127
Carrot Hummus 56
Cashew Cream 143
Celebration Cake 101
Chocolate Cherry Pie 122
Cinnamon Rolls 112
Coconut Cream 142
Coconut Sugar Bumps 110

Creamy Lemon Poppy
   Seed Dressing 51
Eggless Salad 34
Eggless Salad Sandwich 71
Falafel Patties 37
Falafel Salad 36
Fiesta Salad 39
Flax Balls 111
Fruit Cream Cheese 148
Fudge Sickle 114
Ground Meatless 57
Guacamole 59
Hazelnut Bagels 135
Hazelnut Drink 23
Herbed Almond Spread 58
Herbed Cream Cheese 148
Hibiscus Drink 17
Honey Butter 147
Irish Moss Gel 150
Italian Dressing 52
Kale Hummus 55
Kale Strawberry Salad 43

159

Lemon Bars 117
Lemon Pie 108
Lemon Rice 67
Mediterranean Buckwheat Salad 47
Mexican Mind Meld 21
Mint Brownies 116
Mint Shake 18
Mississippi Mud Pie 124
Nancy's Bread 134
Old Fashioned "Potato" Salad 41
Parsnip Chowder 27
Pâté 57
Peach Mint Lemonade 20
Peanut Butter Bars 115
Pizza Crackers 136
Raspberry Lemon Cake 102
Rejuvelac 24

Sauerkraut 60
Sesame Crackers 138
Smart Cat Salad 35
Snapin Carrot Juice 22
Spicy Cheese 146
Spicy Jicama Fries 64
Stawberry Ice Cream 118
Strawberry Dressing 51
Strawberry Frosty 19
Strawberry Kiwi Salad 50
Strawberry Pie 123
Stuffed 'Eggs' 92
Sunflower Beans 56
Sweet Kale Cheesecake 104
Tahini 152
Tahini Sauce 152
Vegan Feta Cheese 149

Summer Recipe Index

Almond Delight 86
Almond Mayo 143
Almond Milk 142
Almond Sour Cream 144
Anytime Breakfast Burrito 80
Arugula Pesto 151
Baja Pulled Eggplant Burrito 90
Banana Date Kebabs 129
Basic Seed Cheese 145
Baykon 87
Bean Burrito 75
Black Bottom Coconut Bars 113
Blond Ambition 114
Brazil Nut Burger 74
Broccoli Crunchy 141
Buttered Zucchini 93
Candied Kale 110
Carrot Brownies 116
Carrot Ginger Cookies 127
Carrot Hummus 56
Cashew Cream 143
Celebration Cake 101
Chocolate Cherry Pie 122
Chocolate Dipped Ice
    Cream Sandwich 120
Chocolate Ice Cream 119

Coconut Cream 142
Coconut Sugar Bumps 110
Collard Herb Rolls 71
Cool Cucumber Soup 28
Corn Bread 132
Creamy Lemon Poppy Seed Dressing 51
Eggless Salad 34
Eggless Salad Sandwich 71
Falafel Patties 37
Falafel Salad 36
Fiesta Salad 39
Flax Balls 111
Flora's Albanian Salad 44
Frosty Drink 19
Fruit Cream Cheese 148
Fudge Sickle 114
Greek Salad 50
Green Zoodles 92
Ground Meatless 57
Guacamole 59
Hazelnut Bagels 135
Hazelnut Drink 23
Herbed Almond Spread 58
Herbed Cream Cheese 148
Hibiscus Drink 17
Honey Butter 147

Impossible Zucchini Pie 97
Irish Moss Gel 150
Italian Dressing 52
Kale Hummus 55
Kale Strawberry Salad 43
Lasagna 76
Lemon Bars 117
Lemon Pie 108
Lemon Rice 67
Mango Smoothie 18
Mediterranean Buckwheat Salad 47
Mexican Mind Meld 21
Mexican Vegetable Soup 33
Mint Brownies 116
Mint Shake 18
Mississippi Mud Pie 124
Moroccan Buckwheat Salad 40
Nancy's Bread 134
Nancy's Peruvian Cheese 144
Open Face Tomato Bites 70
Party Dip 53
Pâté 57
Peach Mint Lemonade 20
Peanut Butter Bars 115
Philly Wrap 73

Pizza Bites 83
Pizza Crackers 136
Raspberry Lemon Cake 102
Rejuvelac 24
Sauerkraut 60
Scrambled Corn Salad 45
Sesame Crackers 138
Simple Salsa 53
Snappy Vegetables 63
Spicy Cheese 146
Stawberry Ice Cream 118
Strawberry Dressing 51
Strawberry Pie 123
Stuffed Anaheim Peppers 65
Stuffed 'Eggs' 92
Stuffed Tomato with Cabbage Salad 46
Sunflower Beans 56
Sweet Kale Cheesecake 104
Sweet Summer Soup 26
Tabbouleh Smoothie 24
Tahini 152
Tahini Sauce 152
Tuna Salad 48
Vegan Feta Cheese 149
Vegetable "Noodle" Soup 31

Fall Recipe Index

Almond Delight 86
Almond Mayo 143
Almond Milk 142
Almond Sour Cream 144
Anytime Breakfast Burrito 80
Apple Carrot Muffins 131
Arugula Pesto 151
Baja Pulled Eggplant Burrito 90
Banana Date Kebabs 129
Basic Seed Cheese 145
Basil Citrus Juice 22
Baykon 87
Bean Burrito 75
Beet Hummus 54
Black Bottom Coconut Bars 113
Blond Ambition 114
Brazil Nut Burger 74
Broccoli Crunchy 141
Broccoli Soup 32

Brussels Sprout Hazelnut Salad 49
Buttered Zucchini 93
Candied Kale 110
Carrot Brownies 116
Carrot Ginger Cookies 127
Carrot Hummus 56
Carrot Mushroom Stir-fry 59
Carrot Raisin Salad 37
Cashew Cream 143
Celebration Cake 101
Chamomile Lemonade 16
Chocolate Dipped Ice
    Cream Sandwich 120
Chocolate Ice Cream 119
Cinnamon Rolls 112
Coconut Cream 142
Coconut Sugar Bumps 110
Collard Herb Rolls 71
Cool Cucumber Soup 28

Corn Bread 132
Cravin' Mac & Cheese 79
Creamy Lemon Poppy Seed Dressing 51
Dirty Rice 69
Eggless Salad 34
Eggless Salad Sandwich 71
Eggplant Kebabs 96
Falafel Patties 37
Falafel Salad 36
Fiesta Salad 39
Flax Balls 111
Flora's Albanian Salad 44
Frosty Drink 19
Fruit Cream Cheese 148
Fudge Sickle 114
Gingerbread Cookies 128
Greek Salad 50
Green Zoodles 92
Ground Meatless 57
Guacamole 59
Hazelnut Bagels 135
Hazelnut Drink 23
Herbed Almond Spread 58
Herbed Cream Cheese 148
Hibiscus Drink 17
Honey Butter 147
Impossible Zucchini Pie 97
Irish Moss Gel 150
Italian Dressing 52
Kale Hummus 55
Ketchup 151
Lasagna 76
Lemon Bars 117
Lemon Pie 108
Lemon Rice 67
Mediterranean Buckwheat Salad 47
Mexican Mind Meld 21
Mexican Vegetable Soup 33
Middle Eastern Marinated Eggplant 78
Mint Brownies 116
Mississippi Mud Pie 124
Mom's Apple Pie 106
Moroccan Buckwheat Salad 40
Nadhirrah's Jalapeño Poppers 66
Nancy's Bread 134
Nancy's Peruvian Cheese 144
Nutty Pumpkin Balls 94
Old Fashioned "Potato" Salad 41

Open Face Tomato Bites 70
Parsnip Chowder 27
Party Dip 53
Pâté 57
Peach Pie 107
Peanut Butter Bars 115
Philly Wrap 73
Pizza Bites 83
Pizza Crackers 136
Pumpkin African Stew 29
Pumpkin Candy 125
Pumpkin Parfait 126
Rejuvelac 24
Rye Bread 133
Salsa 59
Samosa 84
Sauerkraut 60
Scrambled Corn Salad 45
Sesame Crackers 138
Shepherd's Pie 88
Simple Salsa 53
Smart Cat Salad 35
Snapin Carrot Juice 22
Snappy Vegetables 63
Spicy Cheese 146
Spicy Jicama Fries 64
Sprouted Kamut Salad with Vinaigrette 42
Stuffed Anaheim Peppers 65
Stuffed 'Eggs' 92
Stuffed Tomato with Cabbage Salad 46
Sunflower Beans 56
Sweet Kale Cheesecake 104
Tabbouleh Smoothie 24
Taco Meat 57
Taco Salad 39
Tahini 152
Tahini Sauce 152
Tangy Tomato Dressing 52
Tuna Salad 48
Vegan Feta Cheese 149
Vegetable "Noodle" Soup 31
Vegetable Pocket 84
Vegetable Soup Base 31
Veggie Crackers 137
Warm Mexi-Rice 70
Watermelon Strawberry Drink 25
Wild Jambalaya 68

Winter Recipe Index

Almond Mayo 143
Almond Milk 142
Almond Sour Cream 144
Anytime Breakfast Burrito 80
Banana Date Kebabs 129
Basic Seed Cheese 145
Basil Citrus Juice 22
Bean Burrito 75
Black Bottom Coconut Bars 113
Blond Ambition 114
Brazil Nut Burger 74
Broccoli Soup 32
Brussels Sprout Hazelnut Salad 49
Candied Kale 110
Carrot Brownies 116
Carrot Ginger Cookies 127
Carrot Hummus 56
Carrot Mushroom Stir-fry 59
Cashew Cream 143
Celebration Cake 101
Chocolate Dipped Ice
    Cream Sandwich 120
Chocolate Ice Cream 119
Cinnamon Rolls 112
Coconut Cream 142
Coconut Sugar Bumps 110
Corn Bread 132
Cravin' Mac & Cheese 79
Creamy Lemon Poppy Seed Dressing 51
Dirty Rice 69
Eggless Salad 34
Eggless Salad Sandwich 71
Falafel Patties 37
Falafel Salad 36
Flax Balls 111
Frosty Drink 19
Fruit Cream Cheese 148
German Chocolate Donuts 100
Gingerbread Cookies 128
Ground Meatless 57
Guacamole 59
Hazelnut Bagels 135
Hazelnut Drink 23
Herbed Almond Spread 58

Herbed Cream Cheese 148
Hibiscus Drink 17
Honey Butter 147
Irish Moss Gel 150
Italian Dressing 52
Kale Hummus 55
Lemon Bars 117
Lemon Pie 108
Lemon Rice 67
Mint Brownies 116
Mississippi Mud Pie 124
Nancy's Bread 134
Nutty Pumpkin Balls 94
Old Fashioned "Potato" Salad 41
Parsnip Chowder 27
Party Dip 53
Pâté 57
Peanut Butter Bars 115
Pizza Bites 83
Pizza Crackers 136
Pumpkin African Stew 29
Pumpkin Parfait 126
Rejuvelac 24
Rye Bread 133
Samosa 84
Sauerkraut 60
Sesame Crackers 138
Smart Cat Salad 35
Snapin Carrot Juice 22
Spicy Cheese 146
Spicy Jicama Fries 64
Sprouted Kamut Salad with Vinaigrette 42
Stuffed Anaheim Peppers 65
Stuffed 'Eggs' 92
Sunflower Beans 56
Sweet Kale Cheesecake 104
Taco Meat 57
Taco Salad 39
Tahini 152
Tahini Sauce 152
Vegan Feta Cheese 149
Vegetable Pocket 84
Vegetable Soup Base 31

About the Author

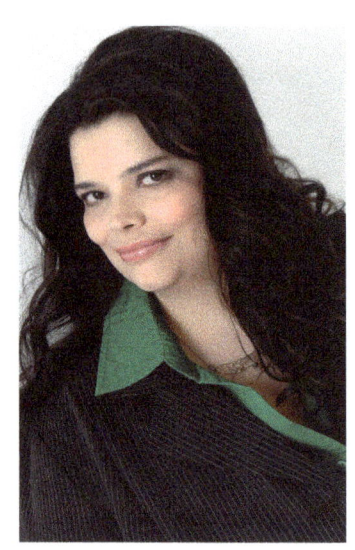

Kachina Choate is a long-time vegetation who ironically, didn't like vegetables. She stood up one day and said "I'm tired of eating food that tastes like twigs, weeds and styrofoam. There has to be a better way." Since then she has been creating and serving healthy food to her unsuspecting friends who when they find out what they have eaten say "I can't believe I ate something healthy... and liked it!"

She is the author of In the Season Thereof, 101 ½ Raw Zucchinis and What to do With Them, Pumpkins Do Grow on Trees, Thriving on Plant Based Food Storage and Kachina Summer Bear Recipe Card Collection.

She began her natural, unprocessed, raw food journey in 2002, and as a result has recovered from depression and kicked a pernicious sugar addiction. She loves to travel and teach healthy food that tastes good.

She started Summer Bear Life Balance Education, a non-profit organization to help people achieve health and a balanced life.

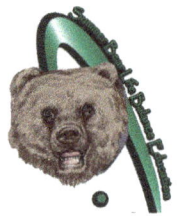

Website: SummerBear.org

Facebook: SummerBearLifeBalance

Instagram: summer_bear_org

Pinterest:
dollkachina/raw-food-wfpb-food-storage-by-summerbearorg
dollkachina/kachina-summer-bears-raw-foods

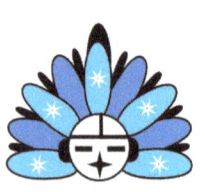

www.ingramcontent.com/pod-product-compliance
Lightning Source LLC
Chambersburg PA
CBHW041128110526
44592CB00020B/2723